ENDORSEMENTS

"Very well done spiritual guide . . . Karen Allen has provided us with an amazing spiritual gift!"

—Edward Partridge, M.D.
Director of the University of Alabama
at Birmingham Comprehensive Cancer Center

"Whether you walk through these pages individually or in a group, your heart will be gripped by the grace only offered through Jesus Christ!"

—Pastor B.R. Johnson
author of *Simple Living in a Complex World*

"Cancer attacks the body, mind, and spirit. Karen has thoughtfully given a spiritual prescription to enable healing of our soul."

—Susan Winchester, M.D.
surgeon

"Good conversational reading style with an upbeat perspective."

—Candy Arrington
author of *Aftershock: Help, Hope and
Healing in the Wake of Suicide*

"*Confronting Cancer with Faith* will walk you through the process of dealing with a life-altering diagnosis through negotiating the small (and large) ignominies encountered in the health care system, interacting with family and friends, working through your thoughts, and waiting for the next test result. This book lets you walk in the shoes of one who has gone before and, while deeply compassionate, places focus squarely on Christ."

—Lawrence Lamb, Ph.D.
brain cancer researcher

"The message of this study is clear: self-examination and faith can serve to help in combating the fear that accompanies a breast cancer diagnosis."

—Lisle Nabell, M.D.
oncologist

To my husband who loves me in sickness and in health. I love you, too, Shug.

CONFRONTING CANCER℞ WITH FAITH

A STUDY OF ENCOURAGEMENT, COMFORT, AND HOPE THROUGH THE TRIALS OF CANCER

Karen O. Allen

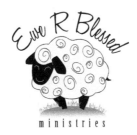

ministries

Published by Ewe R Blessed Ministries, Birmingham, AL. 35242

ISBN 13: 978-1-62480-110-5
ISBN 10: 1-62480-110-2

CONTENTS

PHASE II

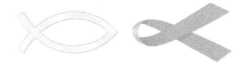

INTRODUCTION

God is bigger than cancer. I was in the midst of chemotherapy for breast cancer when I first heard those words. My hair was falling out, and I was nauseous. The words from my pastor brought a deep sense of reassurance and comfort. Being reminded that God is bigger than what had overtaken my life was exactly what I needed to hear.

Although a Christian for many years, I desperately longed for a deeper connection with God as I endured the trials of cancer. It was time to raise the bar of faith and walk through cancer with courage and strength, giving God the glory.

As I look back on my journey, I realize God had plans for me beyond healing. He wanted me to use my experiences to encourage others going through the same thing. A book would not offer the personal touch and spiritual depth I felt was needed. There should be something more—something interactive, encouraging, comforting, hopeful, educational, biblical, and real. This one-of-a-kind Bible study is written to help meet all of those needs. It is relevant for any person affected by cancer, whether a patient, loved one, or caregiver. My hope and prayers are that it draws you to a closer relationship with God during perhaps one of the most difficult times of your life. Even if you are not a Christian, you will find comfort and empathy from someone who has been through some of the same things you may be going through.

Confronting Cancer with Faith is a six-week Bible study with five lessons for each week. The study covers from the point of suspicion of cancer to remission to possible death. It is divided into three sections: the preparation, the process, and the aftermath. Each lesson takes approximately thirty minutes to complete, inviting your personal involvement. Bible verses from the Old and New Testaments are taken primarily from the New American Standard translation because this was the study Bible my husband gave me years ago. Each lesson opens with a focal verse to introduce the theme. Biblical references and exercises plus reflective questions are intermingled throughout personal insights and stories. A meditative thought is given at the conclusion of every lesson, as well as a dedication usually to someone in the cancer community.

A thoughtful gift of encouragement, *Confronting Cancer with Faith* is a useful tool to guide any person through the trials of cancer at any stage. The study may be used for small groups such as a church setting, a cancer support group, coffeehouse meeting, or for individual study. The primary goal, whether studying in a group or individually at home, is to encourage you to incorporate your "cancer world" into an unforgettable time of spiritual renewal and growth. Using my experience as an example, you, too, can confront cancer with faith while pressing through the fears and uncertainties it brings.

PHASE I

Week 1

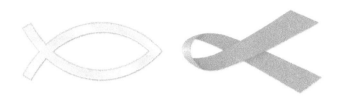

THE PREPARATION: SETTING THE STAGE

When a theatrical play is performed, the stage is set with props, lighting, and back-drops. When cancer is diagnosed, the stage is set with suspicion, anticipation, and fear. But, how will the scene unfold? Who will be among the cast? What script will be followed? The part can be acted out in a number of ways. Focusing on ways that build your faith in God is the most productive. Let's start by recognizing the plot, or purpose in pain. Then, relinquish that pain to the One who desires to suffer along with you and enter into your pain. Plug in to God through quiet time and prayer and lean upon His promises as you prepare to face the trials of cancer. Using God's Word as the script, study it daily as you enter into your new role.

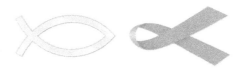

SUSPICION OF THE "C" WORD

Say to those with anxious heart, take courage, fear not . . .

—Isaiah 35:4

It was to have been an unforgettable weekend. Mother had been told months in advance to reserve her birthday weekend and find someone to teach her Sunday school class. The seed of suspicion was planted. As time drew near, Mother's excitement, as well as her suspicions, grew. What was being planned? Where was she going? How should she pack? When the much-anticipated weekend finally arrived, my younger sister, Nancy, drove Mother to my house and decided to tag along as we ventured across town to the house of my older sister, Elaine. Nancy and Elaine contrived to catch a ride with us and be dropped off at the hospital to visit a relative. Nancy's husband, Henry, would then bring them home. *Hmmm . . . a bit odd . . . but OK.* Off we went—the four of us. We were "forced" to divert our route due to traffic, but twenty minutes later with the hospital far behind us, questions surfaced. It was apparent the three sisters were in cahoots! Realizing this, Mother cried tears of joy as her suspicions reached an emotional high. She would be spending the weekend, somewhere, with all three of her daughters—just the four of us, a rare treat. Three hours and two dirt roads later, we pulled into the driveway of a mountain log cabin, and she breathed a sigh of relief.

Saul's Sinister Suspicions

Suspicions—those gnawing inner feelings of uncertainty and wariness. Suspicions can be good or bad. The example of my mother's birthday weekend was a good suspicion; a bad suspicion would be an impending cancer diagnosis. Good or bad, our emotions become elevated and vulnerable in the light of suspicion. Our thoughts become preoccupied, maybe even to the point of obsession.

That's what happened to King Saul. He became obsessed with his suspicions of David. "And the women sang as they played, and said, 'Saul has slain his thousands, and David his ten thousands.' Then Saul became very angry, for this saying displeased him; and he said, 'They have ascribed to David ten thousands, but to me they have ascribed thousands. Now what more can he have but the kingdom?' And Saul looked at David with suspicion from that day on" (1 Sam. 18:7–9). Notice how Saul's suspicions toward David generated emotions of anger and jealousy. That's what suspicions do. They point us toward flaring emotions of doubt, fear, hope, and despair, to name a few. They put us on edge, whether grounded or not.

Suspicions give rise to the need to resolve the conflict within ourselves. For Saul, ending David's life was the only satisfying resolution. He made numerous attempts to kill David and alleviate his perceived threat. The bottom line, as I see it, is that there is a significant need within ourselves to calm our emotional high by eliminating the "unknown element." It takes boldness; it takes tenacity. We desire the truth to be called forth regardless of the outcome.

So what happened to King Saul? Sadly, the Lord departed from him, and he lived in constant fear. At one point, he consulted a medium for advice. Saul relentlessly pursued David but never succeeded in his murderous attempts. Finally, Saul was able to make peace with David through an interesting turn of events. Saul said, "Behold, I have played the fool and have committed a serious error" (1 Sam. 26:21).

Read the story in 1 Samuel 26 of how Saul's suspicions were finally put to an end. What happened that prompted Saul to agree not to harm David?

_____

_____

_____

Although God chose David to one day become king, David recognized God's sovereignty over Saul's life and believed God would remove him from his position in His own perfect time. But, my, oh my, look at the turmoil Saul put himself (and David) through all those years from his jealous suspicions.

A New Year's Surprise

It was January 2003 when I developed a serious suspicion. I say "serious" because I actually had entertained the suspicion three months earlier upon discovering an enlarged lymph node deep in the pit of my left arm. I had felt a twinge of pain a few times, lasting only seconds, prompting my discovery. Even after finding the enlarged lymph node, I dismissed any immediate reasonable course of action, deciding it was nearing the holidays. I would give the swelling a chance to subside—*Nothing much to worry about*, I thought. I'd had an enlarged lymph node before, causing my suspicions to be unnecessarily aroused. I'd even made an appointment with the doctor, but it turned out to be like I had hoped: a swollen lymph node.

Now, after the Christmas holidays, I felt the same twinge of pain under my arm that I had previously dismissed. I inspected the area again, expecting to feel little to nothing; but to my astonishment, not only was the lymph node still there, it seemed like it had gotten bigger! With my suspicions revived, there was the temptation to move to the next level: anxiety. However, my intellect rationalized there was no need to jump to conclusions—yet. I simply needed to schedule that overdue doctor's appointment as soon as possible. I had already promised myself I would call after the first of the year anyway, and now there was no excuse. I took the first available appointment with a request to be called if there were any cancellations.

Looking back on what was later to become a life-changing event, I can see how God used that enlarged lymph node to get my attention and call me to action. It didn't take just one but rather two promptings for me to come to full attention. That is not so unusual for us, is it?

Read 1 Samuel 3:1–10. How many times did it take for Samuel to finally acknowledge God's voice?

_____

You would think Samuel should have recognized God's audible voice, but it took him three times. Samuel finally answered God to tell him he was listening.

There are a number of reasons why we are resistant to God's promptings, among them stubbornness, doubt, busyness, and denial. So, He prompts us again and perhaps again. In my case, I believe God knew it would take substantial evidence to get me to the doctor. Because of the enlarged lymph node, I was compelled to make an urgent appointment. Had I not, the consequences could have been more detrimental in that the undetected tumor in my breast would have continued to grow, just as the lymph node in my arm pit had. The slight pain I felt could have been the infiltration of the tumor draining from my breast into the lymph node, which God thankfully had placed under my arm. For me, a detectable bodily change was required to push me into action. I say "for me" because it is different for each person. For someone else, it may not take a noticeable physical change but rather a hunch that something is not right. A family history of cancer may be enough. For some, it may require a drastic change—such as a golf ball-sized tumor found on a self-exam—to initiate a response. Whatever the severity of the prompt, it is up to us to respond.

How did you or your loved one (if known) respond to the suspicion of cancer?

_____

_____

TO TELL OR NOT TO TELL—NOT A GOOD QUESTION

One thing I did when I first became suspicious of the "C" word was to keep it to myself. Why should I alarm my husband, family, or friends about something that may or may not prove to be true? This was a personal choice. In retrospect, I have to admit keeping quiet was a poor choice because the suspicion raised my emotions to a level where I was almost volatile. I told no one except for a coworker to explain my disappearances from work for medical appointments. Talking to her about my suspicion gave me a slight sense of relief, having shared my burden. "Bear one another's burdens, and thus fulfill the law of Christ" (Gal. 6:2). Any relief I felt, however, was overshadowed by the guilt I had for not having told my husband. I debated for days—months, really—if I should tell Parker of my suspicion until one day God plainly answered my question.

While flipping through an issue of *Guideposts* magazine at home, an article caught my eye. It was entitled "Breast Cancer—Fighting the Fear." Knowing I would be sitting in a doctor's waiting room that afternoon, I grabbed the magazine and headed out the door. As I began reading the article, I was surprised to see it was about a woman's personal struggle in deciding whether to inform her husband of the lump she had discovered in her breast. Imagine that! The article went on to say even though her biopsy was benign, she was relieved to have communicated with her husband in advance. That settled it. *OK, God, I hear You, coming in loud and clear. I will tell Parker.*

I had hoped the message from the article would be twofold: whether to inform my husband and that my biopsy would be benign, like the woman's in the article. That was not to be the case. The message was nothing more than a tangible response to my immediate question of whether or not to inform my husband. It provided me the incentive to press through my strong will and tell the person whom I love more than any other of what was going on in my life. I wondered how best to do this, but I knew God would provide the opportunity.

One evening as Parker and I were dining in one of our favorite restaurants, the conversation shifted, opening a door of opportunity to divulge my suspicion. As I spoke, I simply couldn't bring myself to say the "C" word—that sounded too severe—so, I opted for the word *lymphoma* instead. I tried to minimize the suspicion so as not to trigger alarm. It seemed to work and, whew, was the pressure relieved. Parker received my comments with a different sense of relief, however, saying how my suspicion would explain my recent outbursts of otherwise unexplainable behavior.

Have you ever felt the release of pressure after sharing a suspicion with someone? If so, briefly explain.

_____

_____

_____

FROM SUSPICION TO FEAR

After my confession, my suspicion began to point me to a more intense emotion: fear. Not a paralyzing fear, but a motivating fear. Fear can have different outcomes. On the one hand, it may seem logical to dismiss the fear of cancer, as I did initially since it was nothing more than a self-diagnosis accompanied by a nagging suspicion. On the other hand, the fear of cancer can overcome you to the point of debilitation, preventing you from fully functioning at work, home, or anywhere else. It is understandable to be acutely concerned. It is, of course, much better to allow the fear of cancer to motivate you into constructive action. Do you wait, do you deny it, or do you choose to pursue an answer? If you wait or deny, it could be costly. If you pursue, then you must confront the fear head on.

What kind of fear—paralyzing or motivating—did you or your loved one experience with the suspicion of cancer?

_____

God's Word has a wonderful prescription to combat the grip of fear. "For God has not given us a spirit of fear, but of power and love and discipline" (2 Tim. 1:7). My hope is that as you participate in this study, you will put those qualities of power, love, and discipline God has given you into action.

Meditative Thought

What do you think should be the Christian's response to the suspicion of cancer?

This lesson is dedicated to the memory of Linda Miles, a former coworker who was a dedicated employee of the University of Alabama at Birmingham (UAB) Comprehensive Cancer Center. She never suspected her colon cancer until it was too late. If you or someone you know has a suspicion of cancer, please don't wait and hope it will go away. Make a doctor's appointment today.

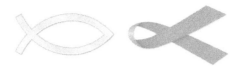

PREPARATION FOR THE JOURNEY

Commit your works to the Lord, and your plans will be established.
—Proverbs 16:3

Ah, the journey, the road toward a much-awaited end, the pathway to a final destination. Where will the journey take us? How will we get there? Will there be stops along the way? "Set up for yourself roadmarks, place for yourself guideposts; direct your mind to the highway, the way by which you went" (Jer. 31:21).

When I think of a journey, I think of an extended, planned adventure—not a short trip or getaway. I also think about who will be traveling with me. In the journey through cancer, trials become our journey companions, teaching us lessons along the way. They navigate our course as we strive to reach the reward awaiting us at the end. What is the reward? A second lease on life or an exercise in faith and character building? Maybe it's a deepening of existing relationships or the renewal of lost ones. Whatever it is, you can be sure when this journey ends, a new one will begin with a new starting point, a new destination, and a new reward. Every journey prepares you for the next.

FAITH: THE DRIVING FORCE

I have heard it said that you are either in crisis, just out of one, or about to go into one. The day you or your loved one was diagnosed with cancer, a journey began. You may be on it right now, or yours may be over. For some, it may be a time of preparation for a journey yet to come. What can you do to make the most of this unwanted journey? How can you be assured of a significant reward at the end? Let me tell you how. Allow the cancer journey to become a journey of faith. That's right. Let this be an opportunity to grow spiritually like you've never grown before.

Avery Willis, co-author of *On Mission With God: Living God's Purpose for His Glory*, says, "When God puts you in a situation that calls for preparation, you can be sure He has already equipped you to handle it by His grace."[1] It has been said many times that wherever His will takes you, His grace will protect you. Begin now, today, to rethink cancer as a journey of faith. It will redefine your outlook and perspective. I promise.

How will you define your journey? Be honest with yourself.

_____   I do not see cancer as a journey with any possibility of reward.

_____   I am not facing this journey now, but I want to be prepared if I do.

_____   I am not ready to face this journey and need some help.

_____   I want to make this cancer journey a journey of faith.

_____   I don't want to think about it right now.

Hopefully, you are ready to deepen your faith through this cancer adversity. If so, it is going to require much discipline. If you are not ready to deepen your faith, at least you made the commitment to participate in this Bible study. If you are not facing this journey and simply want to learn more about cancer and how to deal with it, this study will provide ways to help you offer understanding and support.

BIBLICAL JOURNEYS

A purposeful journey does not come without preparation. The Bible has numerous examples of individuals who went on a journey and how they prepared for it. Consider the journeys of Mary and Joseph before the birth of Jesus (Luke 2:1–7) and later to the temple in Jerusalem for the first time with their son (Luke 2:40–51). There is also the passage of the Good Samaritan, whose compassion was displayed on the road to Jericho (Luke 10:30–37). Perhaps one of the most preached about journeys is that of the prodigal son that led him back into his father's arms (Luke 15:11–31).

Paul's missionary journeys are recorded throughout the New Testament (Acts 13–21) but one of the most well-known journeys of all is the mass exodus of the Hebrew slaves (Israelites) out of Egyptian bondage. God spent eighty years preparing Moses for this great mission (Ex. 1–20). How? Let's look at some ways.

Describe how Moses was being prepared for the Israelites' journey.

Exodus 2:1–10 _____

Exodus 2:11 _____

Exodus 3:1 _____

The first passage refers to Moses' life being spared and brought under the care of Pharaoh's daughter. Not only did Moses learn Hebrew history and culture from his own birth mother who was hired into Pharaoh's household, but he was given the best possible education available from the mighty nation of Egypt. The second passage shows how Moses was aware of the Israelites' oppression on a personal level, and the third passage demonstrates Moses' knowledge of the wilderness. After fleeing what some consider to have been an attempted revolution, Moses took refuge in the desert for forty years as he shepherded his father-in-law's flocks. It was during this time that he learned every detail of the

Midian and Sinai deserts. All of these experiences ultimately prepared him for his great exodus out of Egypt.[2]

A RETROSPECTIVE REVIEW

When I first considered how God prepared me for cancer, I could see, in retrospect, His long-term and short-term preparations. One way was that I worked in a cancer research laboratory at the time of my diagnosis. I helped conduct clinical trials and saw firsthand the heartbreak of cancer and the desperate attempts for longevity of life. I felt the frustration of failed treatment attempts for patients with whom I developed a special fondness, and I witnessed the effects of cancer on families and friends.

When I worked in the laboratory at a Catholic hospital in Louisiana soon after graduating from college, I remember wondering how cancer patients who came to have their blood drawn could be so kind and pleasant. I avoided asking the question, "How are you today?" for fear of their answer. It couldn't be good. They had cancer! I could not understand how these patients faced life so bravely in the midst of such trauma. Why would they possibly care about having a casual conversation with me as I was about to stick a needle in their arm for the umpteenth time? How did these patients find the strength and courage to get out of bed every day and face the world? As the months rolled by, I bonded with the cancer patients from whom I drew blood and began looking forward to their clinic visits. They gave me inspiration. I could see their zeal for life, yet I couldn't comprehend it.

God also seemed to prepare me at strategic points throughout my journey of faith through the use of relevant book studies. One month before receiving my cancer diagnosis, I participated in a book study entitled *Secrets of the Vine* by Bruce Wilkinson. It spoke of how God prunes us for a greater yield of fruit, and how to use that fruit for His kingdom's purpose. "Every branch in Me that does not bear fruit, He takes away and every branch that bears fruit, He prunes it, that it may bear more fruit" (John 15:2). I deeply desired a more productive yield, but that would require more faith than what I had. I prayed for increased faith, believing God would honor that prayer. He did. Of course, it was not in a way I would have chosen. "To this end also we pray for you always that our God may count you worthy of your calling, and fulfill every desire for goodness and the work of faith with power; in order that the name of our Lord Jesus may be glorified in you, and you in Him" (2 Thess. 1:11–12).

> I prayed for increased faith, believing God would honor that prayer. He did.

In the midst of my cancer treatments, David Jeremiah's book *My Heart's Desire* gave wonderful insights on worship which nourished my need and helped me maintain my focus. Last, Linda Dillow's book *Calm My Anxious Heart* gave me the reassurance I needed at the conclusion of my treatments as I approached the telltale mammogram. The book helped me learn better how to live without the crippling fear of cancer recurrence. "Blessed is the man who trusts in the Lord and whose trust is the Lord. For he will be like a tree planted by the water, that extends its roots by a stream and will not fear when the heat comes; but its leaves will be green, and it will not be anxious in a year of drought nor cease to yield fruit" (Jer. 17:7–8).

Aside from my mental and spiritual preparations, my physical body was also prepared. Several months before my diagnosis, a friend and I joined a weight loss program. I lost weight and learned more about proper nutrition. My iron level, which usually hovered below normal, was healthy, and my weight was well within the acceptable range for my height. My immune system had always been robust, but now it was at its peak.

During the time I had become suspicious of the lump under my arm, I wanted to talk to my friend, Jean. She was nearing the end of her radiation treatments for early-stage breast cancer. She seemed to be tolerating it remarkably well. I didn't know how to approach her with my innocent questions without revealing my suspicion. I craved an in-depth conversation with her, not just the "how are you?" kind. God soon made a way. "Is anything too difficult for the Lord?" (Gen. 18:14).

One evening Parker and I saw Jean and her husband, Boyd, at a local seafood restaurant. They were treating themselves to fried oysters. They invited us to join them, affording me the perfect opportunity to ask my probing questions. Jean couldn't quit talking about how good she felt, and I was astounded by the fact that she had gone to the fitness center following her radiation treatment that day. Without ever knowing, she encouraged me with every word she spoke and was a visible example of God's grace. I thought that if she could manage her cancer that well at sixty-plus years old, then I could too—if I had to.

Following my OB/GYN visit, I began to notice how God's peace was being infused into my being as if preparing me for some great challenge. Even with a repeat mammogram, there was no panic. By the time I was to meet with a surgeon for a biopsy and discussion of the results, I was almost expecting them to be positive. Still, I needed to know God was in control. I opened my Bible to Job the morning I would be receiving my pathology report that afternoon. Certainly Job knew about God's steadfastness in troubled times. Chapters 38–39 leaped out to me with great clarity, reminding me that God was not only in control of me but of the entire universe. "Where were you when I laid the foundation of the earth? Who set its measurements? Or who enclosed the sea with doors, when, bursting forth, it went out from the womb; when I made a cloud its garment, and thick darkness its swaddling band, and I placed boundaries on it, and I set a bolt and doors, and I said, 'Thus far you shall come, but no farther; and here shall your proud waves stop'?" (Job 38:4–5, 8–11).

Do you believe God is in control? If so, what evidence do you see?

_____

_____

The words of my favorite hymn "He Leadeth Me! O Blessed Tho't," written by William Bradbury in the 1800s, puts God's role of leadership and our position as followers in perspective.

He leadeth me! O blessed tho't! O words with heav'nly comfort fraught!
Whate'er I do, where'er I be, Still 'tis God's hand that leadeth me!

(Chorus)
He leadeth me, He leadeth me, By His own hand He leadeth me:
His faithful foll'wer I would be, For by His hand He leadeth me.

Sometimes 'mid scenes of deepest gloom, Sometimes where Eden's bowers bloom,
By waters still, o'er troubled sea, Still 'tis His hand that leadeth me!

And when my task on earth is done, When, by Thy grace, the vict'ry's won,
E'en death's cold wave I will not flee, Since God thro' Jordan leadeth me!

PREPARATIONS PROLONGED

A loving aspect of God's leadership and grace is that He continues to prepare us throughout our lives for what is to come. Christian recording artist Rita Springer says she recognized God's intervention early on in preparing her to be a worship leader.

> I started singing in my church and other small churches within the area. Looking back, I realize that the Lord—through my music and circumstances—was already preparing me to minister to others.[3]

I, too, could see how God was preparing me not only for cancer but beyond. There were times I could only look far enough ahead to know that God was in control, but I did not need to look any further. "Do not fear, for I am with you; do not anxiously look about you, for I am your God. I will strengthen you, surely I will help you, surely I will uphold you with My righteous right hand" (Isa. 41:10).

I believe God is preparing each of us for what lies ahead, whatever that may be. "And the Lord will continually guide you, and satisfy your desire in scorched places, and give strength to your bones" (Isa. 58:11).

Meditative Thought

Do you believe God has prepared you for this cancer journey you may be on? If so, how?

This lesson is dedicated to my sweet friend and breast cancer survivor, Cindy Darnell, whose faith remained steadfast and strong through a preparatory time in her life before God blessed her and her husband, Scott, with a miracle baby in the midst of her cancer.

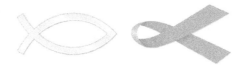

PURPOSE IN PAIN

*For I consider that the sufferings of this present time are not worthy
to be compared with the glory that is to be revealed to us.*

—Romans 8:18

Pain—the gift nobody longs for, still it comes."

These words from the song "In the Waiting," recorded by Greg Long, stir up questions. Gift? Pain—a gift? Is that possible? In the award-winning book *The Gift of Pain: Why We Hurt and What We Can Do About It*, Dr. Paul Brand regards physical pain as one of the human body's most remarkable design features. After witnessing the devastating effects of having no pain sensation, he says if he could choose one gift for his leprosy patients, it would be the gift of pain.

If that's not confounding enough, guess what? Not only is pain a gift, it is a privilege! Jesus said, "For you have been given not only the privilege of trusting in Christ but also the privilege of suffering for him" (Phil. 1:29 NLT). So what is it about pain and suffering that makes it a privilege? Can there be purpose in pain? Yes. Is there purpose in your pain? There can be.

My best friend, Susan Moore, has lived with chronic pain for years. She has learned to befriend pain with courage, perseverance, and faith. She quips, "Somebody has to be me." Susan is a tower of strength and uses prayer as a powerful outlet. Unlike Susan, most of us are prone to ask questions of why, what, and how when difficult times come our way. The truth is we may never know the answer. "Just as you do not know the path of the wind and how bones are formed in the womb of the pregnant woman, so you do not know the activity of God who makes all things" (Eccl. 11:5).

God may not necessarily be at the root of our tribulation but He may allow it. There is a difference. Either way, we must exercise faith and trust to accept that God will not allow anything to come into our lives outside of His will. "Therefore, let those also who suffer according to the will of God entrust their souls to a faithful Creator in doing what is right" (1 Pet. 4:19). Charles Spurgeon said, "Let us put full trust in our Leader, since we know that, come sickness or health, His purpose shall be worked out, and that purpose shall be pure, unmingled good to every heir of mercy."[4]

UNDERSTANDING THE WHYS

God is not accountable to us. However, there is nothing wrong with asking why—as long as we don't get the idea that God owes us an answer. Christ Himself asked, "Why hast Thou forsaken Me?" (Matt. 27:46). If the Lord told us why things happen as they do, would that ease our pain? As believers, we live on promises anyway, not on explanations. Anne Graham Lotz, daughter of evangelist Billy Graham, offers a fresh response to the whys of life. She says, "If you're asking God 'Why have you allowed this?' with the desire to find His purpose so that you might fall in line with it and bring Him glory—I think He is waiting for us to ask questions like that. Sometimes He doesn't show us, but still we should trust Him." [5] She continues by saying she needs to be reminded over and over that she doesn't have to understand. Neither do we; we just have to trust that whatever comes our way, God will bring us through it.

Kim McLaurin of Harpersville, Alabama, couldn't agree more. Her compelling words of testimony at a local Women's Prayer Conference are proof. When she was diagnosed with multiple sclerosis as a young wife and mother, she rationalized that if God wanted her to be healed, He never would have allowed her to have the disease. *There had to be a reason*, she thought. She knew what the Bible said. "For He inflicts pain, and gives relief; He wounds, and His hands also heal" (Job 5:18). Kim prayed God would give her understanding. One day she met a woman and her five-year-old child in an elevator. She learned the woman had recently been diagnosed with multiple sclerosis. Kim shared her source of strength and the woman made a profession of faith, sealing her eternal destiny right then and there. Kim found purpose in her disease, saying she had developed multiple sclerosis so that a woman and her child would find eternal life.

GOD USES OUR PAIN

You've heard it said: there's no gain without pain. The Bible describes numerous instances involving pain. Most precede a blessing. A common reference is that of a woman in labor. Without the pain of labor, there would not be the blessing of a precious newborn. The question to ponder, then, is how do we work through the pain to get to the gain? Let's consider five ways in which God uses pain to bring about gain.

1. **He directs us.** Pain has the ability to move us in a new direction, perhaps toward a new mission or ministry. John Walsh, a recognized television personality whose young son was abducted and murdered, channeled his pain into helping countless families reunite with their missing children while at the same time, placing criminals behind bars. Corrie ten Boom is someone else who was redirected. She never planned to be captured and confined within the barbed walls of a Nazi concentration camp, yet God used her, and still uses her wrenching testimony to convert the cold-hearted, teach forgiveness, and demonstrate love and mercy. "Do not fear what you are about to suffer. Behold, the devil is about to cast some of you into prison, that you may be tested, and you will have tribulation ten days. Be faithful until death, and I will give you the crown of life" (Rev. 2:10).

2. **He inspects us.** What do problems reveal about you? The tea bag analogy applies. If you want to know what's inside a tea bag, drop it into hot water. The same is true for people. When pain

comes into our lives, we find out what is hidden deep within. Another analogy is the refinement of gold. As heat intensifies during the refining process, the deeper impurities surface to create a dross that must be skimmed away. There are times when God is working in us and the hurt that results is bringing out things in us that could only come out under pressure. It is in those times when we learn valuable lessons we would not learn any other way. "In this you greatly rejoice, even though now for a little while, if necessary, you have been distressed by various trials, that the proof of your faith, being more precious than gold which is perishable, even though tested by fire, may be found to result in praise and glory and honor at the revelation of Jesus Christ" (1 Pet. 1:6–7).

3. He corrects us. Some lessons we learn through failure. Anne Graham Lotz suggests that God may postpone His intervention to allow us time to exhaust every other possible avenue until we finally realize without doubt or reservation that we are totally helpless without Him. In those instances, pain turns us back to the Father. "For those whom the Lord loves He disciplines" (Heb. 12:6).

4. He protects us. At a breakfast meeting before Super Bowl XL, Indianapolis Colts Coach Tony Dungy spoke about his son Jordan. He told how Jordan, who has a rare congenital condition, would reach into a hot oven with his bare hands and pull out a pan of cookies. He would burn both hands and his tongue as he joyfully devoured the freshly baked cookies, never feeling a moment of pain. Coach Dungy learned through his son that pain can be used to prevent us from being harmed, sometimes by something more serious. In other words, God may permit us to suffer to keep us away from sin. "You meant evil against me, but God meant it for good in order to bring about this present result" (Gen. 50:20).

5. He perfects us. As Christians, we are called to make a difference in this world and it is often through suffering. Trials build muscles of fortitude allowing pain to serve as a character builder. "We also exult in our tribulations, knowing that tribulation brings about perseverance; and perseverance, proven character; and proven character, hope" (Rom. 5:3–4). Following the release of his film *The Passion of the Christ*, Mel Gibson boldly stated in a PrimeTime™ television interview, "Pain is the precursor to change. That is great news."[6] Really, why is that great news? Because pain and suffering is where glory is found. Reread the focal verse at the beginning of this lesson. We will look at this again in more detail later.

Do you feel God may be using your pain in one of the five ways described above? If so, which one(s) and how?

_____

_____

_____

Pain not only offers us a chance to grow through character and faith, it also offers us a means of realization to expose our weaknesses. Pain has the potential to prepare us for greater work. P.T. Forsyth, a British theologian, said, "It is a greater thing to pray for pain's conversion than its removal."[7] That hits me hard.

Two verses in 1 Peter describe how we should suffer and what our reward is:

> For this finds favor, if for the sake of conscience toward God a man bears up under sorrows when suffering unjustly. But if when you do what is right and suffer for it you patiently endure it, this finds favor with God. For you have been called for this purpose, since Christ also suffered for you, leaving you an example for you to follow in His steps.
>
> —1 Peter 2:19–21

> Beloved, do not be surprised at the fiery ordeal among you, which comes upon you for your testing, as though some strange thing were happening to you; but to the degree that you share the sufferings of Christ, keep on rejoicing; so that also at the revelation of His glory, you may rejoice with exultation.
>
> —1 Peter 4:12–13

What is your initial reaction upon reading these two verses? Think about how you will choose to respond with your or your loved one's pain and suffering.

_____

_____

_____

GOD ENTERS OUR PAIN

Sympathy and compassion are similar but have one major difference: sympathy expresses sorrow from the vantage point of looking from the outside in, while compassion expresses sorrow looking from the inside out.

Which do you think God expresses?_____

The word *compassion* in Latin means "with suffering." "For if He causes grief, then He will have compassion according to His abundant loving-kindness" (Lam. 3:32). The way God views our sorrow from the inside out (compassion) is by entering into our pain. He walks beside us, cries with us, holds our hand, understands our emotions, and knows our heartaches. He captures the depth of our despair, the height of our fear, and the breadth of our concerns because He experiences it right along with us. Hearing that explanation from my pastor brought immediate comfort and relief. *I'm not alone*, I thought. *I can share my cancer with the One who has chosen to enter into my pain with me.*

How does it make you feel, knowing God enters your or your loved one's cancer?

_____

_____

Do you choose to release your pain into His capable Hands? ☐ Yes   ☐ No   ☐ Not Yet

We must be willing to release our pain unto Him to receive the fullness of His blessings. Do yourself a favor—release your pain into God's merciful hands right now.

Meditative Thought

During my cancer treatments, I kept a one-page, colorfully handwritten sheet on my refrigerator given to me by a friend. It encouraged me as I was able to discover the truth of every reason listed and even added a few of my own.

Why God permits trouble or tribulation:

To silence the devil
To glorify God
To make us more like Jesus
To strengthen our faith
To purify our lives
To bring rewards
To teach us patience
To make us sympathetic
To separate us from the world
To make and keep us humble
To teach us to pray
To expand our praise

This lesson is dedicated to my best friend, Susan Moore, who can find the silver lining in any gray cloud. Her loving support throughout my cancer and continued prayers on my behalf inspire me as she endures her own incredible gift of pain.

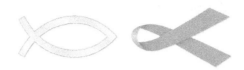

GET PLUGGED IN

*Give attention to my words . . . for they are life to those who
find them, and health to all their whole body.*

—Proverbs 4:20, 22

I have a candid confession. I cannot fathom how anyone can go through the daily grind of life with all of the challenges it brings without Christ at the core of their being. I just can't. "In the day of prosperity be happy, but in the day of adversity consider—God has made the one as well as the other so that man may not discover anything that will be after him" (Eccl. 7:14). How do people find solace through the pain of death or the devastation of cancer without Christ at their side? I have no idea.

If you are participating in this study without Christ in your life, I pray that by the end of these next five weeks you will understand how to fill that empty place by giving your life to Jesus Christ. You do not have to go through this cancer journey, or any other crisis, alone. But more than that, you do not have to go through life alone. You can have the hope and saving grace that only comes from Christ. This lesson, as are the majority in this study, is slanted toward the Christian believer struggling to find victory in Christ through the battle of cancer. However, it is also relevant to the non-believer, who can identify with the elements of victory but may not be able to fully absorb its application.

PREPARING FOR VICTORY

Victory comes with preparation and pursuit, so let's continue together in our preparation for victory over the coming weeks. There is a saying: "The same sun softens butter and hardens clay." The same adversity causes some to succumb and some to become stronger. Which will you choose? I suggest to become stronger, not in your own strength but in God's strength. It is going to take much effort if you truly want to experience the fullness of God's strength through the personal pain in your life. However, participating in this Bible study is a good start.

My lifelong friend Joyce Peters said, "While I would rather not have difficult times come into my life, I fully believe they can shape us into a person that God can use. During difficult times, there is no sitting on the fence—we either turn to God or away from Him." She's right. Clergyman for the local

Emmaus Walk community, Don Roser, is too.[8] He says, "Anything that happens to us is an occasion to either draw near to God or turn away from Him." Rather black and white, isn't it?

Do you agree with the statement that anything happening to us is an occasion to either draw near to God or turn away from Him? ☐ Yes ☐ No

Which one are you doing right now? ☐ Drawing near ☐ Turning away

Unlocking the Power

Spiritual battles cannot be won without divine intervention. Your relationship with God is the key to experiencing God's power at work through you. The underlying question is: how do you develop the relationship to unlock the power? There are many ways but I will focus on two: a dedicated quiet time and daily prayer.

A quiet time. When Jesus became stressed or needed time alone with His Father, He looked for a quiet place, often retreating to the mountains, the wilderness, or a garden. There He sought His Father's will. There He found refreshment for His spirit, body, and soul. He encouraged His disciples to do the same, and He encourages us to seek the same Father as He and the disciples sought. "The hand of our God is favorably disposed to all those who seek Him" (Ezra 8:22). When we seek Him, God promises we will find Him. "You will seek the Lord your God, and you will find Him if you search for Him with all your heart and all your soul" (Deut. 4:29). One of my favorite verses in Jeremiah says, "And you will seek Me and find Me, when you search for Me with all your heart" (Jer. 29:13). Notice the common requirement for finding God in the verses from Deuteronomy and Jeremiah.

What is the key to the search?

_____

The key is to search with "all your heart." Only then will you find Him. Not only does He encourage us to seek Him with all our heart, but He rewards us when we do. "He who comes to God must believe that He is, and that He is a rewarder of those who seek Him" (Heb. 11:6). Now who doesn't like a reward?

So where or how does the search begin? It begins during a quiet time. Seeking God through a quiet time is not the same as a spur-of-the-moment communication which can occur any time throughout the day. A quiet time is an intentional, planned, private meeting—an appointment, if you will—with the Lord God Almighty. There are at least three elements in an effective quiet time:

1. reading the Bible
2. meditating on what you have read
3. praying

A quiet time is a time in which we learn more about God. Reading and meditating upon His Word not only teaches us but brings us hope. "Through perseverance and the encouragement of the Scriptures we might have hope" (Rom. 15:4). A quiet time should also include development of a love relationship with God. "Love the Lord your God with all your heart, and with all your soul, and with all your mind, and with all your strength" (Mark 12:30). As a cancer patient it may be hard to love with all your strength when your strength has faded. In fact, you may feel you have no strength at all; you are doing well just to breathe! If that's the case, then love the Lord with every breath that is within you.

A time for prayer. If we were honest, I bet most of us would admit our prayer lives are best when our circumstances are desperate. That's a start to be sure; but we need to make it a goal to have prayer as a first response in every instance, not a last resort. After all, "He knows the secrets of the heart" (Ps. 44:21).

What are the secrets of your heart right now concerning your or your loved one's cancer?

_____

_____

_____

"Cast your burden upon the Lord, and He will sustain you" (Ps. 55:22). The Lord will do one of two things when you cast your burden upon Him: either remove your burden or provide divine intervention and support. While we probably would prefer the former, it is often through divine intervention and support that God develops our character. It is necessary for our character to match the task at hand or, in this case, the cancer journey to be made. His Spirit works in and through us to produce spiritual growth and character, transforming us more into His likeness. And when we are more like Him, we are less like us.

What do you consider to be the main purpose of prayer? Why do you pray?

_____

_____

_____

In his Bible study *The Prayer of Jesus: Living the Lord's Prayer*, Ken Hemphill says prayer is not about answers or manipulation. It's not about alerting God to our needs. He already knows them. It's not about making us feel better or more peaceful. Nor is it about having our requests granted. Prayer may include some of these things, but prayer is ultimately about rewards—rewards you can enjoy every time you pray. Hemphill says, "God's reward is reserved for those who seek His heart, not His attention."[9] That certainly gets my attention. When I find myself saying, "Help me understand," I have to quickly change it to, "Lord, help me accept." I cannot begin to understand all of God's ways; we aren't expected to, but I do desire to seek His heart.

"Pour out your heart like water before the presence of the Lord" (Lam. 2:19). A very important aspect of prayer is that it must not only be a time of pouring out your heart before God, but you must provide ample opportunity for Him to respond. Pause to recognize God as if in a conversation. This is hard at first and may feel awkward, especially without audible feedback; but this is crucial as you tune yourself in to God to listen for His responses.

One way of getting to know God is by asking questions. God never condemns inquiry. He uses inquiry to teach us. Try it. You expect an answer when you ask a question to a person, don't you? Be mindful, however, that God's answers are often completely different from ours. In fact, even His questions are greater than our feeble answers. "Oh, the depth of the riches both of the wisdom and knowledge of God! How unsearchable are His judgments and unfathomable His ways!" (Rom. 11:33).

Once you have fine-tuned the communication process of talking and listening to God, you will discover that God speaks, guides, and responds. His voice becomes clearer and clearer as you develop an intimate relationship with Him. As your relationship grows, you may find yourself communicating with Him throughout the day. God wants to participate in this cancer journey with you; but in order for Him to actively do that, He needs to be invited.

Will you invite Him to participate? ☐ Yes ☐ No

Why or why not?

_____

_____

A LOOK AT GOD'S GRACE

Even with the self-discipline of daily prayer and a quiet time, there is a hidden link. Without the necessary and vital ingredient of God's grace, these acts are meaningless. The word *grace* in Greek is *charis*, meaning "a gracious favor or benefit bestowed." God's grace is the same for everyone, regardless of church affiliation, employment status, income, or health. Shelia Walsh, Christian author, singer, and speaker, said, "Whether you are spared the battle or you receive the news you most dread, God's grace is the same."[10] Not only is God's grace the same for all, but it is sufficient and powerful. "My grace is sufficient for you, for power is perfected in weakness" (2 Cor. 12:9). Read that verse again. "Grace" and "power" are used in the same sentence as if they are synonymous. I like the fact that God does not render our weaknesses useless but instead uses them to perfect His power through us.

In the song "I Will Run to You" by Darlene Zschech, our pursuit is made plain:

> I will run to You
> To Your words of truth
> Not by might, not by power
> But by the Spirit of God.
> Yes, I will run the race
> 'Til I see your face
> Oh, let me live in the glory of Your Grace.[11]

You may be asking yourself, *If grace is free, then why do I need to pursue it?* Because it is in the pursuit where we find the truth and the perfection of His power, loved one. It's the race that must be run and kept on a steady course until you see His face.

You begin at the starting line. You set the pace. You don't have to be fast or seasoned. You don't have to be poised or refined. All you need to do is put on the proper attire (Bible reading, prayer, quiet time) and start running. "I press on to reach the end of the race and receive the heavenly prize for which God, through Christ Jesus, is calling us" (Phil. 3:14, NLT).

Where do you think you are in your race right now toward the goal of the heavenly prize? (Place an "X" on the line below.)

_____Beginning _____End

It doesn't really matter where you are in the race, just as long as you are in it. Starting the race is an act of faith all by itself. You don't have to have a lot of faith. A little will do. You may feel as though you don't have any faith at all right now, but God is still faithful. "If we are faithless, He remains faithful; for He cannot deny Himself" (2 Tim. 2:13). He is the one who gives us faith to lead us to total dependence on Him.

I am touched by the faith of David Baker, a great trombone player who developed mouth cancer. He said, "On the way up, I called on God for help so why would that change on the way down?"[12] What a tremendous statement of faith. We don't all have that kind of faith; but like Mr. Baker, I have learned that putting my faith into action does not have to feel good. It may feel right but not always good. It is part of the outward expression of my love toward God known as obedience. My former pastor Tom Caradine said, "Obedience is a prerequisite of faith, not a result of it." Be obedient; start the race. You can finish victoriously.

Meditative Thought

You read the statement that your relationship to God is the key to experiencing God's power at work through you. What kind of relationship do you have? Are you ready to see God's power at work through you?

This lesson is dedicated to the memory of my first and last hospice patients, Albert Chambers and Alma Jane Eisenhardt. Alma stayed "plugged in" throughout her illness, adding to the kingdom wherever she was. We shared many prayers together. I did not have an opportunity to get to know Albert before he succumbed to lung cancer, but I have enjoyed a lasting friendship with his wife, Bertha Mae Chambers, better known to me as GrandMae.

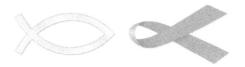

REMEMBERING GOD'S PROMISES

Let us hold fast the confession of our hope without wavering,
for He who promised is faithful.

—Hebrews 10:23

One thing I have discovered during times of great trial is that I revert back to what I believe and know to be true, to what I can claim as consistent and never changing regardless of any external conflict. Those things are God's promises, His character, His Word, who He is, and what He stands for. The fact that I am His child assures me a place of security where I can demonstrate my faith and trust in His steadfastness and be confident of the outcome, whatever it may be. Never mind how desperate and hopeless my situation may seem, nothing is beyond God's grasp. Christian author Sue Monk Kidd says, "Believing is the creative act that helps unlock the impossible in our lives. How limited the world would be if we confined ourselves and God to the possible."[13] With God all things are possible. "Looking upon them, Jesus said, 'With men it is impossible, but not with God; for all things are possible with God'" (Mark 10:27). What better time to put that belief into practice than right now—especially now.

PROMISES YOU CAN COUNT ON

Among the hundreds of promises God gives us in His Word, three in particular seemed to provide me the most comfort throughout my journey of faith. Identify what those three promises are:

"I am with you always, even to the end of the age." (Matt. 28:20)

_____

"Come to Me, all who are weary and heavy-laden, and I will give you rest." (Matt. 11:28)

_____

"I will go before you and make the rough places smooth." (Isa. 45:2)

_____

God's presence is always with us. When Moses led the Israelites out of Egypt, he asked God to show him the way, fully expecting to receive a set of directions and instructions. Instead, God replied, "My Presence will go with you, and I will give you rest" (Ex. 33:14). In other words, He accompanies us in the journey while directing it, and He promises us rest throughout the process.

The phrase "rest in the Lord" brings solace to me. I put this promise into practice often by choosing not to take any sleep aids throughout my cancer ordeal. I wanted to experience God's gentle touch and the truth of His promise even in my sleep. I did.

Another promise is that God goes before us and controls every facet of our lives and circumstances. This is confirmed by His control of an entire universe. Even the frost of heaven (Job 38:29), the birth of a mountain goat (Job 39:1), and the strength of a horse (Job 39:19) are in God's control. He will surely give thought to you and control your outcome.

Have you ever experienced an incomprehensible peace during times of deep despair and unsettling? Why do you suppose that is? If we choose to exercise our faith and trust in God, believing He will do what He says, He will pour out His perfect peace and fill our restless hearts. "God's way is perfect. All the Lord's promises prove true. He is a shield for all who look to him for protection" (2 Sam. 22:31 NLT).

Describe a time in your life when you have experienced God's perfect peace.

_____

_____

_____

_____

Did you have difficulty answering that question? If so, it may be the ideal time to examine your spiritual barometer. If you want a supernatural peace in your life, then you must have a supernatural trust in God. Not a superficial "I believe God is able to do this or that," but a deep-down belief that "God cares about me, and I can place my burdens on Him and not carry them anymore" kind of belief. How do you develop that? One way is to look for the proof in His promises. Why are the promises there in the first place? It's not because He needs to remind Himself of what He will do for us. It's because we need to be reminded of what He can and will do for us. When we trust God's promises and see the evidence of them in our lives, we come closer to developing the peace and assurance we long to have. But first there are some prerequisites.

PREREQUISITES TO GOD'S PROMISES

God cannot deal with us outside the nature of His character. This is not surprising. Therefore, in order for us to experience the full value of God's promises, there are several basic criteria that must be met. First, you must have faith and knowledge in the promiser. The power to believe a promise depends entirely on your faith in the promiser. Second, you must relinquish your will unto His will. When we pray, we are asking God to let us see the world as He does. God desires for us to actively participate with Him in doing His work, thus providing us an opportunity to quit worrying about our own earthly kingdom as we begin to seek His kingdom. Third, you must position yourself to be in obedience to Him. Henry Blackaby and Claude King, co-authors of *Experiencing God: Knowing and Doing the Will of God* say, "Obedience is the outward expression of your love of God. It shows faith in

Him. The reward for obedience and love is that He will show Himself to you. Affirmation from God will come only after your obedience."[14]

Let's evaluate where you stand. Mark the following prerequisites as having been accomplished in relation to your cancer journey:

_____ I demonstrate faith and knowledge in God (even if it's weak)

_____ I have relinquished my will to His will

_____ I practice obedience to God

If you were unable to check all three, perhaps this will give you a good starting point to do some soul searching. As I have mentioned, having an intimate relationship with God is the single most important thing you can do as a Christian. Of course your health, family, and career are important. Lots of things are important, but nothing is more important than having an intimate relationship with God.

Blackaby and King describe the steps toward having an effective relationship with God: "When you come to a moment of truth when you must choose whether to obey God, you cannot obey Him unless you believe and trust Him. You cannot believe and trust Him, unless you love Him. You cannot love Him, unless you know Him."[15] So let's get to know Him more.

A Peek at Some Precious Promises

We have established that God never has or ever will fail to be whom He promises to be. So what are some of these promises?

Identify God's promise in each of these verses.

Zephaniah 3:17 _____

Isaiah 41:10 _____

Isaiah 43:4 _____

Philippians 4:19 _____

Psalm 91:5 _____

Hebrews 13:8 _____

Proverbs 3:5–6 _____

Isaiah 26:3 _____

While the above list gives only a sampling of God's long list of promises, these verses help demonstrate that you are not forgotten and He sees your plight. The cliché "God promises a safe landing, not a calm passage" may apply. However, a phrase in the chorus "Shout to the Lord" sums it up nicely for me: "Nothing compares to the promise I have in You."[16]

Psalm 23 is a psalm often read for comfort that contains many of God's promises. Below is an adaptation from an unknown source with the insertion of God's promises.

The Lord is my shepherd—That's relationship

I shall not want—That's supply

He maketh me to lie down in green pastures—That's rest

He leadeth me beside the still waters—That's refreshment

He restoreth my soul—That's healing

He leadeth me in the paths of righteousness—That's guidance

For his name's sake—That's purpose

Yea, though I walk through the valley of the shadow of death—That's testing

I will fear no evil—That's protection

For thou art with me—That's faithfulness

Thy rod and thy staff they comfort me—That's assurance

Thou preparest a table before me in the presence of mine enemies—That's hope

Thou anointest my head with oil—That's consecration

My cup runneth over—That's abundance

Surely goodness and mercy shall follow me all the days of my life—That's blessing

And I will dwell in the house of the Lord—That's security

Forever—That's eternity

Identify three of God's attributes found in this beloved psalm that are the most pertinent to you today.

BELIEVE AND RECEIVE

Once you have met all the prerequisites and your beliefs are intact, you are primed. However, there is one more vital step: you must receive. It is one thing to believe God's promises; but unless you receive and validate them by putting them into your everyday living, what application do they have? Without application, you are being deprived of God revealing Himself in a real and personal way. If you haven't already done so, start believing, receiving, and seeing God achieve His promises in your life. Accept the promises of peace and comfort through your current trials by establishing and putting those beliefs into action. Let your trust serve as the glue between believing and receiving. "For all the promises of God in Him are Yes, and in Him Amen, to the glory of God through us" (2 Cor. 1:20 NKJV).

Meditative Thought

We see evidence of God's promise to Noah when we look in the sky at a rainbow. Which of God's promises are evidenced in your life?

This lesson is dedicated to Karen Ott, a sweet friend, spiritual mentor, and longtime survivor of cervical cancer. She walks daily with joy in God's promises, inspiring others as she delights in His Living Word.

Week 2

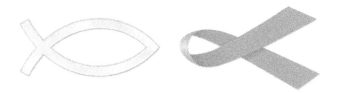

THE PROCESS:
THE DIAGNOSIS

Now that we have set the stage, we are ready to tackle the difficult process of dealing with cancer. Over the next four weeks we will look at the cancer process, incorporating four primary components: the diagnosis, the plan, the effects, and the responses. Lessons concerning the diagnosis will look at different kinds of tears, the emotional and physical impact, recognition of authority, the value of support systems, and the significance of a broken spirit. Open your heart and let me walk with you through "The Process" of cancer.

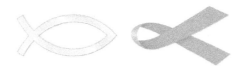

A TIME TO CRY

I am weary with my sighing; every night I make my bed swim,
I dissolve my couch with my tears. For the Lord has heard the voice of my
weeping, the Lord has heard my supplication, the Lord receives my prayer.
—Psalm 6:6, 8–9

Every cancer patient knows the day of his or her diagnosis. For me, it was Friday, January 31, 2003. It was a day that started off much like any other as I readied myself for work. All morning I kept busy before Parker came to pick me up after lunch to go meet with the surgeon. We would be getting the results of my biopsy.

As we walked toward the surgeon's office, I blurted out that my intuition led me to believe the results were going to be positive. God's preparations for me seemed all too clear. In reality, the statistics were in my favor since the vast majority of all breast biopsies turn out to be benign. I was hoping not to be the "1" of the 1 in 8 women diagnosed with breast cancer in the U.S. every year.[1] I had no family history of cancer and maintained a relatively healthy lifestyle. It was reasonable to believe I would be no different from most other women, but that was not how I felt. God prompted me to say what I was thinking out loud to my husband. Parker asked me why I felt my results would be positive and then he affirmed his love for me. Those few words were some of the sweetest words I had ever heard as he tenderly spoke of my character, my personality, and my spirit being what he loved, not just my physical body. I knew all of that but it felt good to hear it. It gave me an opportunity, too, to hear his reaction as I considered what it might be if it were medically necessary for me to have a mastectomy. My announcement also gave Parker a chance to absorb the possibility of what was soon to become reality.

As we tried to relax in the crowded waiting room, my anxiety level began to climb. I had been able to occupy my thoughts at work but now I was still and contemplative. I spotted a Bible on one of the corner tables and began reading it to once again occupy my mind. Immediately, I turned to the book of Psalms and reread Psalm 139—the passage Dr. Susan Winchester had suggested I read the day before. It was apparent why as I reread it.

Read Psalm 139. Why do you think this psalm was suggested for me to read at the time of my biopsy?

_____

_____

The Office Couch

As the minutes dragged into an hour, my anxiety turned to agitation as I thought of how cruel it was to make someone wait so long to find out if their life was about to be changed forever. Of course, other lives were being impacted, too—not just mine. So, I read psalm after psalm before turning to Psalm 119, the longest psalm in the Bible. Surely by the time I finished reading that psalm we would be called back, but no. As I turned to yet another psalm, I knew I was not absorbing a word of it; but I rationalized that at least I was filling my mind with the Word of God. Finally, Parker and I were ushered to the couch in the surgeon's office. I determined this was a bad sign. Dr. Winchester sat down and methodically retraced the steps that had led us up to this point. She reviewed the mammogram and ultrasound reports and then presented the biopsy results. As Parker and I squeezed each other's hands, my palms now sweating and heart pounding, Dr. Winchester revealed the results. They were as I had thought, just as God had prepared me: positive. Parker and I did not gasp or act overwhelmingly alarmed but simply sat there in a state of subdued shock. *Positive.* My results were positive. Working in the medical field and having encountered many oncology patients, I had wondered what the scenario was like for both the doctor and the patient. Now I knew.

Dr. Winchester stepped out of her office to allow us a chance to absorb the devastating news. She later returned to describe the surgical options available to us. As she explained what "moderately differentiated ductal in situ carcinoma" meant and then began drawing diagrams and discussing alternatives, I realized this was way more than I was ready to digest. *Positive*—I was still stuck on that. Not only did I have cancer that was ten minutes old, but now we were being told we would have to make a decision as to what we felt was medically, personally, and spiritually best for us. It was no longer in the surgeon's hands but rather in our laps! Why didn't Dr. Winchester just tell us what to do so we could do it? Why couldn't the choice be clear-cut? Should we elect the most conservative approach (a lumpectomy) or the most radical and comprehensive approach (a double mastectomy)? My head was spinning. I tried to focus on the discussion, but I heard only parts of it as *positive* still rang in my ears.

At the end of the explanations, I glanced over at Parker, whose eyes were now red with flowing tears. I had been able to keep it together fairly well, I thought, up until that point. But now sadness gripped my heart to see his lips quiver and face wrinkle, trying to hold back the intense sorrow he was feeling. After twenty-plus years of marriage, I knew him well enough to know it was not a selfish sorrow but rather a selfless sorrow. It was impossible for Parker to displace this horrible reality by sacrificing himself, which he gladly would have done. He knew that I, alone, would have to endure the physical aspects of what was to come. Worst of all, there would be pain and discomfort. But as one, we would face it together.

Wouldn't you guess that God must have wrestled with similar feelings, knowing His only Son, a part of Himself, would be mercilessly hung on a cross after unimaginable suffering and pain? Yet, this was the only way—the only way to forgive the sins of the world through the perfect sacrifice of a perfect Lamb. "He Himself is the propitiation for our sins; and not for ours only, but also for those of the whole world" (1 John 2:2).

For me, Parker's tears of sorrow translated into greater love. But for the world, there is an even deeper and further-reaching love that is given to us through Jesus' death and resurrection. Parker's desire was to ease my suffering and offer comfort; I wanted to soothe his hurting heart. The best I could do at that moment was join him in crying.

Keenly sensing our desire for spiritual intervention, Dr. Winchester took each of our hands as we made a small circle. She prayed for us right there on her office couch. What a feeling of compassion, reassurance, and godly intervention there was in that one act of uncharacteristic behavior in an uncharacteristic place from a godly physician servant.

BACK TO WORK

We left the doctor's office and Parker took me back to work at my insistence. On the drive back, I felt a deep sense of oneness with Parker as I assured him I would be OK despite any pain that might be involved. This seemed to be of great concern to him. Upon returning to work, the only person who knew where I had been phoned to ask about the results. I told her. I knew I would have to tell my boss and other coworkers, too. One coworker had been through the biopsy process with his wife just a few months earlier, but her results had turned out to be negative. It had been an anxious moment for our "lab family," and I wondered then why I had taken such a strong interest in Joseph's wife's situation. Now it was plain to see: God used her to help set the stage for me.

When I saw Joseph, I began to tremble as tears welled up in my eyes. It was much more difficult to divulge my secret through a face-to-face conversation than it had been to answer a question over the phone. I prefaced my words with, "Remember when your wife had that biopsy and her results came back negative? Well, mine didn't." I choked as I came upon the dreadful "C" word, feeling as if it were being extracted from my mouth.

Those would not be the only tears I would cry in the coming months. There would be many more: tears of grief, despair, anger, fear, shame, and of the unknown. But God took those tears and worked a small miracle in my heart. He turned my tears to tears of joy, faith, worship, sacrifice, and praise.

TEARFUL TIMES

In the book of Ecclesiastes, Solomon ponders God's sovereign design, concluding that all events in life are divinely appointed. "There is an appointed time for everything. And there is a time for every event under heaven, a time to weep, and a time to laugh; a time to mourn, and a time to dance" (Eccl. 3:1, 4).

I would like to propose three categories of tears. These are not categorized by an emotional response but rather by purpose. The categories are:

1. God's call *for* tears
2. Our response *in* tears
3. His response *to* our tears

The category in which we most frequently find ourselves is number 2 "our response *in* tears." God's compassion is moved by our tearful responses, which brings greater purpose to our tears. But there are times when God actually calls us to cry perhaps to bring recognition of our wrongful acts, leading us to seek forgiveness.

Below is a list of verses representing one of the three categories of purposeful tears. Mark the following verses as 1, 2, or 3: God's call for tears, our response in tears, or His response to our tears. Some verses may have more than one category.

_____ "Arise, cry aloud in the night at the beginning of the night watches; pour out your heart like water before the presence of the Lord." (Lam. 2:19)

_____ "Blessed are those who mourn, for they shall be comforted." (Matt. 5:4)

_____ "When she opened it [the basket], she saw the child, and behold, the boy was crying." (Ex. 2:6)

_____ "Thus says the Lord of hosts, 'Consider and call for the mourning women, that they may come; And send for the wailing women that they may come!'" (Jer. 9:17)

_____ "He will swallow up death for all time, And the Lord God will wipe tears away from all faces." (Isa. 25:8)

_____ "And standing behind Him at His feet, weeping, she began to wet His feet with her tears, and kept wiping them with the hair of her head, and kissing His feet, and anointing them with the perfume." (Luke 7:38)

_____ "In the days of His [Jesus] flesh, He offered up both prayers and supplications with loud crying and tears to the One able to save Him from death, and He was heard because of His piety." (Heb. 5:7)

_____ "Those who sow in tears shall reap with joyful shouting." (Ps. 126:5)

BOTTLED UP TEARS

There are really no wrong and right answers for this exercise. What is most important is that all of our tears belong to God. One of my favorite verses, Psalm 56:8, says, "Thou hast taken account of my wanderings; put my tears in Thy bottle." I love this verse because it tells me God is attentive to every detail of my life, down to saving the tears that fall from my eyes. I imagine a bottle filling higher and higher each time I cry. I would only hope God's bottle for me is big enough!

Not long before my diagnosis, my friend Sharon gave me a beautiful bottle as a gift. I had once shared with her this verse and my sentiments about it when she was going through a difficult time. The bottle she gave me was a smooth-cut, stain-colored glass with a chipped glass stopper. It may have been a perfume bottle at one time. I asked Sharon where she found it. She confessed it came from a pawn shop making it all the more special to me. I symbolized its correlation to Jesus' simple origins of life to death: a borrowed manger to a borrowed tomb. To me, the bottle's beauty came from its origin, the marred stopper, its significance, and the one who gave it to me. I use the bottle to collect oil from special anointings. It is one of my greatest treasures. It reminds me that God knows and understands what I am going through and how I feel.

Meditative Thought

Do you have a special treasure that reminds you of God's thoughts about you? If not, consider creating one. An example might be a painting of a beach in which the grains of sand represent God's thoughts concerning you or a bird singing songs as God sings over you.

This lesson is dedicated to the memory of Susan Marchase, an administrative director in the Department of Medicine at UAB. Susan received the Outstanding Woman UAB Faculty Member award in 2002 before succumbing to cancer in 2004. The Susan D. Marchase Outstanding Woman Administrator Award was created in her memory for women demonstrating leadership, vision, courage, dedication, a commitment to the university, and advancement of women in the community. As the 2006 recipient of this prestigious award, I desire to fulfill my continued commitment toward the worthwhile goals set before me.

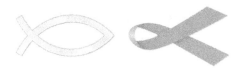

THE WHIRLWIND BEGINS

When my spirit was overwhelmed within me, Thou didst know my path.
—Psalm 142:3

Have you ever noticed when disasters strike they bring with them an unsympathetic and indiscriminate to-do list? The immediate aftershocks following a disaster stir up an unexpected whirlwind, spinning us 'round and 'round until it finally stops, leaving us breathless and dizzy. There is no denying—the whirlwind is real. It is unavoidable, unrelenting, and all-consuming.

What is a whirlwind anyway? According to *Merriam Webster's Collegiate Dictionary*, it is "a small rotating windstorm of limited extent; a confused rush; a violent or destructive force or agency."[2] Let's adapt that definition to look at it from a different perspective. For the newly diagnosed cancer patient, a whirlwind is an accelerated pace of life involving a maze of doctor appointments; medical tests; frequent hospital, clinic, and pharmacy visits; confusing medical terms; mind-boggling decisions; schedule rearrangements; work adjustments; lengthy phone conversations; sleepless nights; and hours of reading and research. And that only scratches the surface. It doesn't come close to describing the sudden overwhelmed feeling one experiences during the whirlwind do-this, do-that period.

As you might expect, looking upward into a whirlwind's rotating funnel results in tunnel vision. My tunnel vision could be described as a temporary, apathetic attitude toward the rest of the world's affairs apart from my own. For example, I usually like to send cards of encouragement, support, or commemoration to family, friends, and church members, but that seemed an impossible task in light of my circumstances. Another example was my surprising postponement of compassion and sympathy toward a national disaster in which several people lost their lives. This tragedy occurred the day after my diagnosis, but I wasn't able to concern myself with such things. I was in my whirlwind period. Even after the initial whirlwind period, I didn't turn on the car radio for months. It seemed too worldly, too intrusive, and irrelevant. I either drove in silence or listened to an instrumental CD.

THE EMOTIONAL WHIRLWIND

At first, the whirlwind seems almost as equally encompassing as the disaster itself. That's because the whirlwind contains the list of immediate things which must be attended, things that become a non-stop blur of action. I view this as the physical element, the visible whirlwind. It eventually completes its course, usually lasting but a few weeks. However, the greater, more powerful, and potentially destructive element of the whirlwind is the one that cannot be seen. That is the emotional whirlwind. It must be soothed and tamed with gentle strokes of patience and conscious acts of discipline. The emotional whirlwind cannot be satisfied with the physical fulfillment of checking off a to-do list. It must be dealt with on a more personal level. The emotional whirlwind doesn't have a definitive time frame like the visible whirlwind; it can last for months, even years.

Parker and I received my diagnosis on a Friday afternoon, allowing the shock to be absorbed over the weekend. At my surgeon's advice, we opted not to make any decisions about surgery until we'd had a chance to talk it over and sift through our thoughts. We spent a quiet weekend at home with our dogs. Saturday night, Parker took me to a nice Italian restaurant. When Sunday came, we attended church as usual. I filled my seat in the choir loft and Parker counted the first-of-the-month Sunday offerings. It appeared on the outside to be as any other Sunday in the Allen household. However, that was far, far from the truth. At my request, we kept the news of my cancer to ourselves until I had a chance to inform family and close friends. Plus I wanted to soak in the last Sunday of being "normal" before being "converted" to a cancer patient.

Rather than subsiding, the emotional whirlwind grew more turbulent for Parker over the next few weeks. His mother's increasing health needs diverted his attention. My mother-in-law, who lived forty miles away, had been hospitalized for several weeks, and now Parker and his sister, Cindy, faced the difficult decision of whether or not to move her into an assisted-living facility. Meanwhile, my own emotional whirlwind was in full rotation as I experienced a widespread gamut of emotions: fear, relief, anxiety, peace, sadness, trust, apprehension, disbelief, acceptance, grief, and love, to name a few. Life as I knew it had ceased, and now I had to find a way to cope with this new "thing." Although Parker and I were both enmeshed in our own personal emotional whirlwinds, we shared common ground, finding solace in one another.

What emotions have you felt during an emotional whirlwind? It may be about something other than a cancer diagnosis.

_____

_____

How did you handle those emotions?

_____

_____

A BIBLICAL BLOW-BY-BLOW

God knows exactly the kind of human whirlwinds we endure. Look at the description given in Proverbs 1:27–28: "When your dread comes like a storm, and your calamity comes on like a whirlwind, when distress and anguish come on you, then they will call on me."

It may surprise you to discover how frequently whirlwinds are mentioned in the Bible. First of all, we see that God orchestrates whirlwinds and displays His sovereignty in them. "Before your pots can feel the fire of thorns, He will sweep them away with a whirlwind, the green and the burning alike" (Ps. 58:9).

God also used whirlwinds in specific ways such as,

to scatter: "Thou shalt winnow them, and the wind shall carry them away, and the whirlwind shall scatter them; and thou shalt rejoice in Jehovah, thou shalt glory in the Holy One of Israel" (Isa. 41:16).

to give a descriptive comparison: "Its arrows are sharp, and all its bows are bent; the hoofs of its horses seem like flint, and its chariot wheels like a whirlwind" (Isa. 5:28).

to bring calamity: "But I will kindle a fire in the wall of Rabbah, and it shall devour the palaces thereof, with shouting in the day of battle, with a tempest in the day of the whirlwind" (Amos 1:14).

and to spare a prophet from death: "Then it came about as they were going along and talking, that behold, there appeared a chariot of fire and horses of fire which separated the two of them. And Elijah went up by a whirlwind to heaven" (2 Kings 2:11).

My favorite way of how God used whirlwinds is seen in the following two verses.

"Then the Lord answered Job out of the whirlwind." (Job 38:1)

"The sound of Thy thunder was in the whirlwind." (Psalm 77:18)

What is the common denominator for these verses?

God is always in the midst of the whirlwinds. Isn't that amazing? Doesn't that bring you comfort? Like Job, He will speak to you out of your whirlwind. Hopefully it will not be like thunder, but you can be sure He is speaking. Will you hear Him? In order to hear, you must listen, which requires you to set aside time from your chaotic to-do list and discipline your out-of-control emotions. Only then are you more apt to discern His voice and receive His comfort.

That's not all. Not only does God orchestrate the whirlwind, is in the midst of it, and speaks out of it, but His way is found in it. "The Lord is slow to anger and great in power, and the Lord will by no means leave the guilty unpunished. In whirlwind and storm is His way, and clouds are the dust beneath His feet" (Nah.1:3).

Wait. There's more. You'll be glad to know that the whirlwind has a limited lifespan like the Webster definition says. It will eventually pass. Notice the word *when* in this verse: "When the whirlwind passes, the wicked is no more, but the righteous has an everlasting foundation" (Prov. 10:25).

Which aspect of the whirlwind described above do you most relate and why?

_____

_____

Let's recap. We have learned that God orchestrates and displays His sovereignty in the whirlwind, He is in the midst of our own personal whirlwind, He speaks to us through it, His way may be found in it, and the whirlwind will end.

Let me leave you with one last thought. Chariots are mentioned numerous times in conjunction with the whirlwinds God sent (Isa. 5:28, 2 Kings 2:11, Isa. 66:15, Jer. 4:13, and Dan. 11:40). Remember the song "Swing Low, Sweet Chariot?" I like to envision God sending His chariot deep into my whirlwind to symbolically invite me to be His passenger. The chariot doesn't have to be taking me "home," but it would certainly provide a glorious ride with a dependable driver holding the reins. Now that's what I call sweet.

Meditative Thought

How will you apply what you have learned today to the whirlwinds of your life?

This lesson is dedicated to the memory of Annette Ramey, a hard working mother who endured more than her share of life's hardships. She faced the end of life with courage and honor before succumbing to brain cancer at an early age.

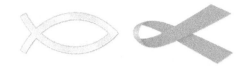

ORDER IN THE TELLING

Encourage the exhausted, and strengthen the feeble. Say to those with anxious heart, "Take courage, fear not."

—Isaiah 35:3–4

After receiving my diagnosis, I tossed around the question of who I should tell. Then I asked myself the question of when and how to tell them. I theorized at one point that perhaps God's glory could best be demonstrated through a display of personal strength by keeping my illness private. My hope was that others, in retrospect, would perceive God's intervention and strength in my life once they learned of my cancer from other sources. After giving it some consideration, however, I rationalized, *Where's the glory in that?* Furthermore, why would I want to deprive myself of the support that could be so readily available to me? The correct answer to my question became obvious. Yes, yes, yes, I should tell. I should tell family and friends so God's glory could be seen through the proclamation of who He was (and is) in my life during my day of trouble, not hidden in my silence. He would shine through me so that others could see. Ah, now that would be a demonstration of God's glory as well as a demonstration of my faith.

With that decided, Parker and I faced the dreaded task of informing family and friends of my diagnosis. I devised a general plan for prioritizing whom to tell, when, and how. This may not be important to some, but it seemed like a sensitive issue to me warranting thoughtful consideration. There was no prescribed right or wrong way; cancer does not come with an etiquette book. Certainly there was no easy way. Nonetheless, it was a plan—an order, if you will. "But let all things be done properly and in an orderly manner" (1 Cor. 14:40).

Identify someone you believe glorifies God. What does that person do to make you think that way?

_____

_____

RECOGNITION OF AUTHORITY

Not only did I want a systematic order to tell the significant people in my life of my cancer, but I wanted it to be reflective of the positions of authority I respected. For example, first came familial authority: husband, mother, sisters, in-laws. Second, was "earned" authority: employer, coworkers, friends; and third, spiritual authority: church staff, deacon body, Sunday school, and church choir.

Jesus recognized His position and assertion of authority based upon His relationship to the Father. "Truly, truly, I say to you, the Son can do nothing of Himself, unless it is something He sees the Father doing; for whatever the Father does, these things the Son also does in like manner" (John 5:19). After John the Baptist baptized Jesus, followed by the descending of the Holy Spirit upon Him, Jesus was led into the wilderness. He was, in effect, "covered" by the Holy Spirit as He faced Satan's temptations. I love what happened after that: "Angels came and began to minister to Him" (Matt. 4:11). I, too, felt ministered to as the pastor and deacon body held a special anointing for Parker and me a few days before my surgery. I felt "covered" by the authority of the Holy Spirit, my husband, and the church leadership.

CATERING THE SHOCK

Apart from the recognition of authority and order, I wanted to approach each person with a catered delivery of my news. I wanted it to be specific to the individual and compatible to their personality. My news would be shocking since there was absolutely no sign of my health ever having been compromised. I was every bit as active as I'd ever been, although my energy level had waned over the last few months. I had told no one of my suspicion save one coworker before finally telling Parker, as you have already read.

I decided to approach my best friend and my boss with hard-core facts. I presented my friend Susan with a copy of my pathology report. She was familiar with such reports, having a medical background and working in a clinic for years. She was also a former Southeastern Conference sports official and liked to know the rules and game plan. As I recalled my steps leading up to the biopsy results, I sensed she was hurt from my not having told her of my suspicion; but she gracefully dismissed my oversight to offer consolation and support. We had been through a lot together with her chronic health issues. Now we would have to confront mine.

As an oncologist, my boss, Dr. Pierre Triozzi, was accustomed to receiving and delivering difficult news, so a positive pathology report was nothing out of the ordinary. What was out of the ordinary was that it had his lab manager's name on it. I'll never forget Dr. Triozzi's unusual response. "This will just be a big inconvenience for you," he said. *Cancer an inconvenience? I'll say!* I wasn't sure whether to be offended or encouraged. How could he minimize something so catastrophic? Maybe it didn't have to be catastrophic. Since he dealt with cancer every day, I decided he knew what he was talking about. I accepted his comments with confident inspiration. Rather than my cancer being catastrophic, it was metamorphic (life-changing). As for being a big inconvenience— well, it was most assuredly that.

> My news would be shocking since there was absolutely no sign of my health ever having been compromised.

Dr. Triozzi graciously offered his professional and medical support. I was fortunate to be able to tap into his wealth of knowledge and experience to confirm decisions and/or ask questions. He offered me medical leave but I declined. I gave him permission to tell my male coworkers so as not to make them feel uncomfortable in my presence. I also asked him to make it clear it was OK to talk about my cancer in the lab. I opted not to inform work associates outside my immediate area so as to maintain as much normalcy as possible for myself as well as for my work environment.

The news to my friend Sharon required a gentler approach. She is much younger than me and needed to hear the news directly from me followed by consolation and reassurance. She would not be as interested in a proposed plan of action at this point. I determined she would take the news the hardest. I had become like a mother and mentor to her after she lost her mother to brain cancer a year earlier. At times Sharon would plead for me never to get cancer, yet here I was disclosing her worst fear. Using spiritual references and an elongated introduction, I began my soft delivery. But in the midst of it, I lost my nerve and ended up making my dreadful news into a guessing game. This was not the gentle approach I had planned—but she forgave me.

Parker acted as my informant for my mother and in-laws. I had asked him not to tell my mother so that I could, but he was scheduled to see both his mother and mine on the afternoon of my "D-day" (diagnosis day). His distraught state begged the obvious question as to what was wrong. Unable to comply with my request, Parker took advantage of the moment and divulged the distressing news. Saddened to tears, Parker and my mother provided each other a kind of support for which my presence would have been intrusive. They needed the opportunity to react freely and uninhibited without the pretense of being strong in front of me. Feeling much relief from Parker's confession of having told my mother, I followed up with a phone call that evening. We spoke at length as I relayed to her that I was OK and asked her to please tell my two sisters so they could, in turn, tell their families the way they felt most appropriate.

Briefly describe two different approaches that you or your loved one used to divulge a cancer diagnosis.

_____

_____

_____

There were still a few others yet to be told. Susan offered to tell some of my other friends so I would not have to repeat the same story again and again. I was most grateful. The monotonous repetition had begun to feel as though it were taking on an impersonal attitude of "let's just get this over with." By the eighth time, it almost seemed to have a detached tone. The whole process was mentally draining. I was ever so glad when it reached the grapevine stage.

As for telling the church, I chose to handle that myself. I started with the church staff by writing a letter to the pastor, asking him to share it at the next weekly staff meeting. I requested that my name be withheld from the prayer bulletin that week so I would have ample opportunity to inform the sanctuary choir, of which I was an active member. I asked the choir director to serve as my spokesperson as I slipped out at the end. By the following week, my Sunday school class was already aware of the news so there was no formal announcement. Also, my name was added to the church prayer bulletin, informing the remaining church membership.

In addition to my family, close friends, coworkers, and church, there were still a few that needed to be informed. These were primarily friends in organizations in which I was involved, plus a few long distance friends. I chose to e-mail this group of individuals. At first I was concerned an e-mail might seem insensitive, but it was well received—so much so that I decided to send out periodic updates. My e-mail updates developed into a diary of sorts of my spiritual journey. The list of recipients grew with each mailing, and I began to get feedback of encouragement and prayerful support from people I didn't even know. I learned that my e-mails were being forwarded to others to serve as inspiration, which humbled me deeply. People even began asking to be put on my e-mail list.

No Offense Intended

As a possible well-meaning, future informant, let me offer two words of caution to you. First, be careful not to overstep your boundaries in terms of spreading the cancer news. I recall the disappointment I felt when I learned that an elderly friend of mine had been told of my cancer by a well-meaning friend. This dear lady had become like a grandmother to me. She was the wife of the first hospice patient for whom I had provided volunteer support. Since I only saw GrandMae, as I called her, on an irregular basis, she would have never known of my cancer had she not been told. Aside from the fact that I was unsure of how she would respond, I thought it might be nice to have one friend who knew nothing about my illness. It would allow me the freedom not to have to discuss how I was feeling that day or how my treatments were going. It may have been selfish, but I wanted just one person with whom I could be "normal." As it turned out, GrandMae was glad to have been told. I, too, was glad, having underestimated her wisdom and strength. However, it is advisable to first ask if it is OK to tell others rather than making that assumption yourself. "Do not be wise in your own eyes" (Prov. 3:7).

Second, don't be offended if you are overlooked in the "got cancer" information hotline. It is likely to have been a simple oversight. It may be hard to imagine how this could happen but it can. In fact, it is rather easy amidst the whirlwind of activity. Understanding goes a lot further than taking offense. "A man's wisdom gives him patience; it is to his glory to overlook an offense" (Prov. 19:11).

Meditative Thought

How would you want to be told of a loved one's cancer diagnosis?

This lesson is dedicated to my medical team of physicians and nurses including Martha Harrison and Drs. Susan Winchester, Lisle Nabell, Pierre Triozzi, and Sharon Spencer. Their expertise, accompanied with compassionate delivery and quality care, provided me with confident direction and healing.

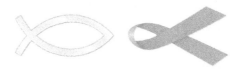

GATHERING SUPPORT

For the eyes of the Lord move to and fro throughout the earth that
He may strongly support those whose heart is completely His.
—2 Chronicles 16:9

There comes a time when pride of independence must be displaced with the comfort and encouragement from others willing to lift us up during difficult days. It took me only a short time to reach the point to willingly submit to the support that was available to me. It was hard to be on the receiving end, as I was more accustomed to being on the giving end. I wanted to retain my stubbornness and deny that I had a serious illness requiring help. I wasn't in pain but who was I fooling? I needed all the support I could get. The truth is, the sooner you accept the love and support from others, the sooner you can settle in to the business of healing.

There are a variety of support systems, many of them unique and specific to individual needs or cancer types. There are support groups through churches and medical facilities. There are cancer organizations nationally and regionally that provide a supportive network. There are cancer websites, blogs, message boards, and chat rooms as well as trained social workers and counselors. You don't have to look far to find support beyond family and friends.

Once the word spread of my cancer, it did not require any effort on my part to glean support. It just happened. News spanned all the way from Birmingham, Alabama, across international borders to Romania. I cannot tell you how many prayer lists I was on, but I can tell you that I was thankful to be on each one of them. You can never have too many people praying for you and offering their support. A fervent commitment to prayer is the best support anyone can give. However, if others don't know about your or your loved one's cancer, they cannot offer support. So don't withhold information and deny or defer support when you need it the very most.

JUST SAY OR DO SOMETHING

One thing in particular I learned through this journey that I never would have understood to the extent I do now. That is, it is vitally important for concerned individuals to acknowledge your or your loved one's cancer in some way. It doesn't have to be involved or time-consuming, like cooking a meal, making a visit, or offering your services. It can be simple, like a phone call, a card, or a kind word such as "I'm sorry to hear of your illness." It can be anything. I'll go so far as to say it can be wrong! Just say or do something. Please. It's painfully obvious when you choose not to acknowledge the elephant in the room for the sake of an awkward moment. Whatever you say or do is appreciated and considered an act of support (as long as you are not prying for information).

As a cancer patient, it is easy to become self-centered and self-absorbed. This is understandable. You are focused upon your needs, your health, and your concerns. There is a natural tendency to become oblivious to the needs of others without realizing it. At first I found myself making excuses not to trouble anyone on my behalf; but what I forgot was that some people, especially those closest to me, felt helpless and needed to do something tangible for me. They needed to feel like they could contribute to my cause. It was enlightening when I finally took a step outside my circle of self-absorption to put myself in their shoes.

Describe a simple act of support (if applicable) that was meaningful to you or your loved one.

_____

_____

_____

I am going to veer from the lesson format this one time to share a brief allegory involving my primary support systems. This is meant to serve as both a resource for support systems you may not have thought about and is also a heartfelt thank-you to those mentioned. I wish I could acknowledge every individual who supported Parker and me, but that is not possible. "And every survivor, at whatever place he may live, let the men of that place support him . . ." (Ezra 1:4).

RESIDENTS (RESIDENCE) IN THE CITY OF HOPE

There is a large community located within the Kingdom of Christ known as the City of Hope. All cancer patients and their families move to this city and live there the rest of their lives. At the heart of the City of Hope is the Well of Living Water operated and controlled by a Father and His Son. This is where the power and water purification plants are found. The Well of Living Water has been there as long as anyone can remember; everything seems to revolve around it in one way or another. The Father, Son, and their partner, Holy Spirit, provide sustenance for all of the residents to meet their daily needs. There's always enough power and water for everyone—not too much, not too little.

The Avenue of Support is the main street running through the middle of the City of Hope. There are many inlets that feed into the Avenue of Support. Among them are Friendship Lane, Church Street, and Club Court. At the uppermost point of the Avenue of Support is Family Circle. That is where my husband and I live along with my mother, my two sisters, Elaine and Nancy and their families, Aunt Ethel Mae, and my cousin, Cathy. My mother-in-law, sister-in-law, Cindy, and her husband, Jerry, live a few blocks away. Family Circle is a close-knit neighborhood. We keep up with the latest news on the street and visit one another as often as possible. My times are never more special than when they are shared within the Family Circle.

Parallel to the Avenue of Support is Medical Parkway. Drs. Nabell, Winchester, and Spencer work there. I see them often since I work in the Cancer Center's Helping Hands Lab across the street. Dr. Triozzi is my boss and the Helping Hands lab director. Dr. Triozzi, Wayne, Joyce, Mark, and I make up the Helping Hands lab team. There are other helpful people on Medical Parkway such as Nurses Martha, Kendra, and Ronda. They gladly share a smile and comforting word to every cancer patient they see.

A short distance from Medical Parkway is Friendship Lane. This is a busy road since lots of people live there including Joyce, Cathy, Marsha, Joanne, Martha, Theresa, and Kathryn. Ever since Parker and I moved to the City of Hope, the residents on Friendship Lane go out of their way to bring us food and gifts. Debbie offered to clean my house once. The two people I see most often on Friendship Lane are Susan and Sharon. Susan is one of those friends you can always count on, especially for dire short-notice needs. Sharon has a way of lifting your spirits whenever you are down.

Near Friendship Lane is Church Street. Parker and I are active members of one of the larger churches on Church Street. We have many friends there like the Campbells, the Moores, the Otts, and the Overstreets. We have friends at other churches, too, like the Johnsons, the Peters, and the Munns. Our church friends are a vital entity of our lives, and we consider them to be a stabilizing force during days of great trial. Pastor Anton, his wife, Elizabeth, and their son, Alex, are a special blessing to us. Pastor Anton gave me a wonderful book upon our arrival to the City of Hope entitled *Words of Encouragement*. He often quotes from this book. I sometimes find myself grasping at his words as they give me renewed strength to press onward. Reverend Randy gave me a precious gift of scented oil I use only for special occasions.

At the intersection of Church Street and Friendship Lane is Mentor Manor. This is, of course, where the Mentors live, Boyd and Jean. They are delightful people and are good friends with the Father, Son, and Holy Spirit. Jean invited me to visit Mentor Manor as soon as she heard we had moved to the City. She and Boyd had moved there a year earlier and knew what it felt like to be newcomers. Jean made herself available to answer all of my questions, even the embarrassing ones. I was grateful for her kindness, particularly the pointers she gave me on what to wear to the upcoming Radiation Ball. She helped me select the best make-up and lotions for my skin type.

Club Court is an interesting neighborhood. It is full of character and personality. Charlene, Dale, and Patty live in Critter Companion Estates. They have a huge backyard with—you guessed it, lots of critters. Charlene runs the store at Canine Corner where my four dogs, Alamo, Frezno, Skippy, and Susie, like to shop and sniff. The dogs enjoy strolling down Club Court, stopping at Med Tech Mansion's mailbox where Linda and Peggy live. They also stop at Susan Komen's country house, too, with its beautiful, fragrant flowers and sculpted bushes that always seem to need "watering." Support Group Square is one mile past Club Court but I never go there. Some of my friends do. They like the shopping and camaraderie.

> It's amazing the amount of power contained in the flock as a whole.

Memory Lane is a fun and exciting place. Sharon, Jimmie, David, Allison, Mary Helen and her son all live there. Parker and I have shared some happy moments on Memory Lane. We love hearing from our friends whenever they call or send a card.

One day as I was traveling down Memory Lane, I heard a loud honking noise in the sky. I looked up to see a flock of geese in a "V" formation heading south for the winter. I had recently learned from my bird-watching class that together the whole flock adds over

70% flying range as each bird flaps its wings to create a supportive uplift for the bird behind it. *How interesting*, I thought. It's amazing the amount of power contained in the flock as a whole. I learned that when a goose falls out of formation and begins to feel the drag and resistance of flying alone, it quickly gets back into formation to take advantage of the power from the flock. As I continued watching, the tired lead goose rotated back and let another goose take the lead. All the while the geese honked as if to encourage the lead goose to keep its momentum. Watching the geese, there was no doubt in my mind that they would make it to their destination. *What a wonderful example*, I thought, *of gathering support. Even the geese understand its importance.*

Around the corner from Memory Lane is a curious street to me: Stranger Alley. People will walk up and begin talking to me as if they know me. I've decided they do this because they see me wearing the same hat they are wearing and want to share with me where theirs came from and how old it is. I like Stranger Alley; I find a sense of bonding there. Oddly enough, I've noticed there's a Stranger Alley in every city where Parker and I go. It astonishes me how many people have the same hat!

With all of the residents in the City of Hope, I am rarely ever alone. But even with the wonderful places and people, the most appealing thing about the City of Hope is the Father, Son, and Holy Spirit. Something about them draws me into their presence. They are always available, keeping their cell phone on all hours of the day and night. I can call anytime and I do. Yes, indeed, I am convinced there is no better place of residence than in the Kingdom of Christ.

Meditative Thought

A Cancer Patient Speaks:

What can you do or say to offer support for me?

Be honest with me. I can tell when your feelings or actions are insincere.

Laugh with me, cry with me. Allow me to express intense emotions.

Don't feel sorry for me. Your understanding helps preserve my dignity and pride.

Touch me. I want to be accepted despite the way I may look. Inside, I'm still the same person you always knew.

Let me talk about my illness if I want to. Talking helps me work through my feelings.

Let me be silent if I want to. Sometimes I don't have much energy and I just want your silent companionship. Your presence alone can be comforting.

Space your visits and calls. Consistent support is very helpful.

Support my family. I may be sick, but they, too, are suffering. Give them an opportunity to express their feelings.[3]

This lesson is dedicated to Jean Jordan, a breast cancer survivor, who mentored me and showed me that cancer can be donned with grace and dignity.

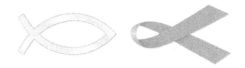

IN THE PLACE OF BROKENNESS

The spirit of a man can endure his sickness, but a broken spirit who can bear?
—Proverbs 18:14

It has been a hard week. First, there was a lost job opportunity. Then my international coworker received word she would have to start her green card process over again. One of my friends received notice that her school tuition was due and there's no loan money left in her account. Sunday, our church hosted a farewell reception for our third staff member to leave in the past two months. And last, my best friend was having her sixteenth foot surgery. No doubt about it, it has been a hard week.

You have read about the processes associated with the diagnosis of cancer this week: crying, a whirlwind atmosphere, informing others, and gathering support. All of these things bring us to the culminating high point of brokenness. That's right, I said brokenness. You might be wondering how that can possibly be a high point. Here's how. It is in the place of brokenness where transformation occurs. God wants to revive and transform our hearts, but it must begin with brokenness and humility—no exceptions, no shortcuts, no substitutions. "I dwell on a high and holy place, and also with the contrite and lowly of spirit in order to revive the spirit of the lowly and to revive the heart of the contrite" (Isa. 57:15).

In the book *Brokenness: The Heart God Revives*, Nancy Leigh DeMoss writes that our culture is obsessed with being whole and feeling good to the point of affecting the way we view Christian life. We want gain without pain, the resurrection without the grave, life without death, and a crown without the cross. But in God's economy, the way up is down and the way to be first is to be last. DeMoss says we will never meet God in revival until we first meet Him in brokenness.[4] I agree. "Humble yourselves in the presence of the Lord, and He will exalt you" (James 4:10).

Abraham Lincoln had his share of brokenness before and after his presidency. He said, "I have been driven many times upon my knees by the overwhelming conviction that I had nowhere else to go." Why must we come to the place of brokenness before dropping to our knees? Do we fall prey to our human nature, feeling the need to exhaust all possible earthly solutions first? Why do we wait so long to finally humble ourselves in utter brokenness before God?

Answer the above questions in a personal way.

_____

_____

_____

BROKEN CARS, BROKEN PEOPLE

Let's get practical. I believe there are four approaches toward something that is broken. The first is to do nothing, allowing the broken item to remain just as it is: broken. This is an easy option requiring no effort, but then it does not address the problem. In fact, the problem will likely worsen the longer you avoid it. Denial does this by delaying acceptance. The second approach is to replace the broken item with a new one. While this will achieve the end result with minimal effort, you still have not addressed the broken item, only replaced it with a substitute. The third and best approach for our purpose is to repair the broken item so that it functions properly once again. This takes time and involves adjusting, realigning, rebuilding, and/or replacing broken parts. It may also require the skills of a specially trained expert.

Let's use the example of a car. When your car breaks down, you do not abandon it on the highway, never to return. Nor do you go out and buy a new one every time it dies. Instead, you attempt to fix Ol' Nellie yourself or take it to a mechanic to evaluate the problem. It is corrected to a renewed condition using the necessary tools and/or parts. Whatever it takes, you pay the price to restore your car to its full operation.

There is a fourth approach to something that is broken. Unlike the other three, it is counterproductive. It involves anger and retaliation. Giving the broken car a good kick on the wheel while speaking your mind is an example. You may feel better temporarily, but it does nothing to repair the car. Plus you end up with a sore toe!

I know it's a stretch, but for illustration purposes let's compare cancer to the broken car. I am referring not only to the physical brokenness but the mental and spiritual brokenness of cancer as well. You can plod through a medical plan to address the physical needs, but have no intention of addressing the mental and/or spiritual needs that require just as much attention. You see no reason to exert more effort to grow and gain something of personal and spiritual value out of this cancer journey. You're tired. You don't feel like doing what it takes to strengthen your faith. Sound familiar? "Be renewed in the spirit of your mind" (Eph. 4:23).

Maybe you are the exact opposite. You overexert yourself, pouring yourself into your work, your hobbies, or your family, hoping your fears will vanish—but they never do. Perhaps the counterproductive approach fits you best, affording you an excuse to be angry with God for "giving" you or your loved one cancer. Please, please let me implore you not to waste your precious time and energy fighting God while you are fighting cancer. "Let us therefore draw near with confidence to the throne of grace, that we may receive mercy and may find grace to help in time of need" (Heb. 4:16).

In which of the four approaches do you see yourself right now? Is this where you want to be?

_____

_____

FROM OUR BROKENNESS TO GOD'S BROKENNESS

Now that we have discussed some approaches to brokenness, let's focus on what spiritual brokenness means. Our idea of brokenness and God's idea of brokenness are two different things. We tend to think of brokenness as being sad—gloomy, depressed, or constantly putting ourselves down. We think of it as an emotional experience accompanied with a continuous flow of tears. But God's definition of brokenness is not like that. It is centered around humility. "The Lord is near to the brokenhearted, and saves those who are crushed in spirit. Many are the afflictions of the righteous; but the Lord delivers him out of them all" (Ps. 34:18–19).

Luke 18 describes two men who went into the temple to pray. One was a Pharisee and the other was a tax collector. The Pharisee stood and prayed, "God, I thank Thee that I am not like other people: swindlers, unjust, adulterers, or even this tax-gatherer. I fast twice a week and I pay all my tithes" (v. 11–12). But the tax collector, unwilling to lift his head, prayed, "God, be merciful to me, the sinner" all the while beating his chest (v. 13). Verse 14 goes on to say, "I tell you, this man went down to his house justified rather than the other; for everyone who exalts himself shall be humbled, but he who humbles himself shall be exalted."

Describe a time in which you felt a deep sense of humility.

_____

_____

_____

True brokenness is an ongoing lifestyle change. It coincides with what God believes should be the condition of our heart. *Contrite* is a word often used in the Bible to indicate a sense of brokenness. Being contrite dismisses self-will and surrenders to God's will. The broken person has no confidence in his own works but rather is totally dependent upon God's grace to work in and through him. Being humble allows us to be more receptive and responsive to the Word of God. "But to this one I will look, to him who is humble and contrite of spirit, and who trembles at My word" (Isa. 66:2). It also sets the stage for transformation: a conversion; a change in condition or character. "But we all, with unveiled face beholding as in a mirror the glory of the Lord, are being transformed into the same image" (2 Cor. 3:18).

IT'S ALL ABOUT TRANSFORMATION

Henry Blackaby and Claude King called it a "crisis of belief" in their *Experiencing God* study. A "crisis of belief" is when you come to a crossroads where you must make a decision about how you will choose to respond, but let's take it a step further. According to Blackaby and King, you can either choose to do something that has God-sized dimensions and be transformed in the process or you can choose not to. It is dependent upon your outlook and attitude. These two things help determine your outcome and reaction.[5]

Are you willing to be transformed with God-sized dimensions in the process of your or your loved one's cancer journey?　　□ Yes　　□ No　　□ I'm not sure

The first time I heard the song "Bring the Breaking" by Casey Corum, I was astounded by the words presenting a plea for brokenness:

> Bring the breaking in me
> Reduce me to love
> Let Your life now be lived through me
> And the walls come down
> Bring the breaking
> Please bring the breaking.[6]

The truth is that nothing could be more pleasing to God than a broken spirit. "The sacrifices of God are a broken spirit; a broken and a contrite heart, O God, Thou wilt not despise" (Ps. 51:17). Being broken does not mean being shattered; it means having the chance to be remade and remolded. In other words, transformed. Martin Luther said, "God creates out of nothing. Therefore until a man is nothing, God can make nothing out of him."

Transformation is a process that takes time and involves unseen events taking place within the heart. This, of course, is God's specialty. It begins with the mind, which is the gateway to the transformation of the heart.[7] "And do not be conformed to this world, but be transformed by the renewing of your mind" (Rom 12:2). In order to be transformed, we must renew our minds every day. It is only when the renewed mind lines up with the heart that we become new creatures, inside and out. Thus, an internal transformation leads to an external difference.

Look at the transformation of the caterpillar into a butterfly. It must go through the difficult process of forcing itself through the chrysalis to mature its wings and become the beautiful new creature it was intended to be. Without the internal transformation, it cannot obtain the exquisite color and perfect shape of its delicate wings that allow it to fly. You may not feel like it, but you can become that new creature. The ugliness of cancer does not have to reside in your heart. Decide now to renew your mind every day so you can begin to transform your internal brokenness into an external glory.

Oh, and by the way, another job possibility opened up, my coworker's green card process looks hopeful, my student friend was given two monetary gifts, our church has reorganized the deacon body to facilitate enhanced unity, and my friend's surgery was a success. What easily could have fostered a spirit of brokenness has now been transformed into opportunity and glory.

Meditative Thought

Identify some broken areas of your life that need transformation and write a statement as to how you are going to address these areas. Allow your brokenness to be the very thing that serves to strengthen you.

This lesson is dedicated to the memory of Mavis Tennyson, a saintly woman who experienced much brokenness in her life due to sickness, sorrow, and life's disappointments. She channeled her brokenness into a faithful witness for Christ, before and during her cancer journey.

Week 3

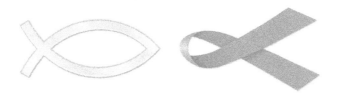

THE PROCESS: THE PLAN

During the second week of "The Process" (third week of study) we will focus on "The Plan" incorporating the implementation of cancer treatments such as surgery, chemotherapy, and radiation. In addition to a medical plan, we will also address a spiritual plan to recognize God's presence and comfort in our lives. It is through the spiritual plan where we draw strength to effectively cope and build our faith through the challenges cancer brings.

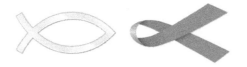

GOD REACHES OUT

I will lift up my eyes to the mountains; from whence shall my help come?
My help comes from the Lord, Who made heaven and earth.

—Psalm 121:1–2

A cancer diagnosis is followed by a plan of action. The plan may be preventive and precautionary, it may be proactive and aggressive, or it may be passive and palliative (hospice care). The plan may involve surgery, chemotherapy, and/or radiation. Or, it may involve symptomatic pain management and comfort with no curative measures. Whatever the plan, the medical team works with the patient and their family to facilitate its effective implementation.

My plan of action involved a combination of aggressive and preventive measures: surgery, chemotherapy, and radiation—the big three. I will refer to this as my medical or treatment plan, addressing each one separately during the course of this week's study. Before discussing the medical plan, however, let me introduce my spiritual plan. Just as the medical team designed a treatment plan to meet my medical needs, God designed a spiritual plan to meet my spiritual needs. Each person's medical and spiritual needs are different, but perhaps my sharing of these plans for me will encourage and inspire you.

GOD USES PEOPLE

When God reaches out, He does so in many ways. One way is through people—lots and lots of people. Divine guidance does not have to exclude humans. God uses people according to their talents and abilities. Consider the surgeon and the oncologist. Others include family, friends, clergy, church members, coworkers, educators, other cancer patients—even strangers. All of these people can be used by God to achieve His purpose.

I have identified four categories of how God used people to reach out to me during my journey of faith. They are: people who brought comfort and encouragement, people who brought healing, people who supplied needs, and people who clarified and/or confirmed decisions. Time and time again, I saw how God used these individuals to meet my immediate, short-term, and, in some cases, long-term medical and spiritual needs.

Identify someone you know in each category who relates to you or your loved one.

Comfort and encouragement: _____

Healing: _____

Needs supplied: _____

Clarify/confirm decisions: _____

Now, let's look at some biblical characters God used to reach out to others. Identify the character and what specific task was accomplished through that individual.

	Character	**Task Accomplished**
Joshua 1:1, 6		
Daniel 2:26–30, 47		
Luke 7:1–10		

Joshua succeeded Moses to ultimately bring the Israelites into the land of Canaan. Daniel was used to interpret King Nebuchadnezzar's dream, and the centurion was used as a vessel of faith to bring about the healing of his sick slave. All of these men were effective in being used by God to accomplish His purpose.

A SLOW DANCE WITH GOD

In addition to using others to reach out, God specializes in unexpected ways of reaching out that only He Himself can do. Overcoming fear and achieving acceptance fall into this category. I never knew there were so many levels of acceptance to be achieved as God reached out to me over and over again. Conquering fear and dread in order to achieve acceptance was an ongoing process throughout my cancer. The example below sounds somewhat trivial now, but at the time I guarantee you it was anything but trivial. For some reason, I was mortified at the thought of having to spend the night in the hospital following surgery. Although I was not scheduled to stay overnight, the possibility existed. I don't know why I could accept the surgery but not an overnight hospitalization. The fear was overwhelming.

One morning after my quiet time, I sat in the easy chair in our bedroom crying. I didn't know how I could be so scared of something that happens to people every day. It was ridiculous. Besides, I was accustomed to the medical environment, having worked in it my entire career. How was I going to overcome this fear? It made no sense.

As my CD softly played, my crying became muffled. I felt as if God had walked into my room and up to my chair. He spoke my name, introduced Himself, and asked me if I would join Him in a slow dance. I was so stunned, I stopped crying. I wondered, *Is this for real? Are you sure?* Not wanting to take a chance on missing an extraordinary encounter with God, I stood up slowly and closed my eyes. I wanted to absorb every second of the moment and, at the same time, not distract myself by my own conspicuous actions. I couldn't help but think how silly I must look as I held out my hands as if to say, *OK, God, let's dance.*

I stood there motionless, drenched in fear as I once again began to sob. *I can't do this, God,* I said silently. *I can't move.* I felt paralyzed.

God quietly whispered in my ear, "You don't have to. Let me. Stand on my feet."

Stand on your feet? Are you sure about that? I queried. *OK then.* As I submitted to His request, I began to gently sway my upper body without moving my feet. As this continued, I felt the fear gradually start to fade. As it faded, my feet began to move ever so slightly from their locked position as I picked them up just inches off the floor. They felt as heavy as bricks as they barely moved while my hands and arms were in full dancing partner position. Soon I was able to take a step as if to follow my partner's lead. *This is it,* I thought. *This is what I need to understand. I need to let Him lead. I have nothing to fear when I follow His lead.* It was a tremendous moment of release and revelation.

As the CD played, I began to tune in to the words being sung: "I'm desperate for you." It was perfect, chosen by God. By the end of the song, we were dancing all around the floor of my bedroom. My tears had subsided, along with my fear, and just like that I was ready to face an overnight stay in the hospital (which God knew would happen).

"People say that God gives you nothing you can't handle, but that's not true. God gives you nothing that you and He together can't handle." Well said, Coach Sammy Dunn, whose faith challenged many high school students before he succumbed to cancer.

Describe a time in which God brought you to a place of acceptance that you didn't have before. Or you might recall a time when you think you might have missed an incredible encounter with God.

_____

_____

_____

A year after my dance with God, I was astounded by an e-mail I received from my older sister Elaine. She didn't realize I had lived what this unknown author spoke about:

> Guidance. While meditating on the word *guidance*, I kept seeing "dance" at the end of the word. Doing God's will is a lot like dancing. When two people try to lead, nothing feels right. The movement doesn't flow with the music, and everything is uncomfortably awkward. When one person realizes that and lets the other lead, both bodies begin to flow with the music. As gentle cues are given, the two become one body, moving beautifully. The dance takes surrender, willingness, and attentiveness from one person and gentle guidance and skill from the other.
>
> When I saw the "G," I thought of God, followed by "u" and "i." "God," "u," and "i" "dance." God, you and I dance. I became willing to trust that I would get guidance about my life by letting God take the lead.

THE CHICKEN LIVER STORY

God's reaching out included not only other people and supernatural intervention, it also included music, His Word, praying, visions, personal and corporate worship, Christian books, symbolism, and reminders of His presence. I will elaborate on some of these throughout the course of this study. Remember, God designed these ways to meet *my* needs, so this list is specific to Karen O'Kelley Allen. Your list will be different. Of course, some of these means (e.g. prayer, His Word, worship) are relevant to everyone.

A humorous example of God's reminding me of His presence occurred one day at lunch. I decided to go across the street to get some fried chicken livers since I had been trying to increase my iron and protein intake during chemotherapy. When I got there, I was disappointed to see none were left. I sauntered back to the hospital cafeteria with a wilted zeal. *How many people seek out chicken livers for lunch?* I wondered. As I stood in line, a fleeting thought popped into my head. *How God-like it would be if the cafeteria were serving beef liver and onions.* This was a common menu item I enjoyed at work. I laughed out loud when I reached the window. Lo and behold, right in front of my very eyes was showcased a steaming pan full of fried chicken livers! In all my years of working at UAB, I'd only seen chicken livers served a few times. I thanked God right then and there for His everyday blessings and for reminding me how much He cared and thought about me, including what I had for lunch. One of my favorite verses in Psalm 139 came to mind. "How precious also are Thy thoughts to me, O God! How vast is the sum of them! If I should count them, they would outnumber the sand" (Ps. 139:17–18).

SEEING THE SYMBOLISM

As mentioned, God reached out to me often through the use of symbolism. Jesus frequently used symbolism when telling parables to illustrate a point. Symbolism is used in the Bible to represent something significant and abstract. For example, animal sacrifices in the Old Testament were representative of forgiveness and appeasement (Lev. 17:11). The Lord's Supper is symbolic for the remembrance of Christ's broken body and shed blood for us (1 Cor. 11:24–25). Symbolism can also represent something with common characteristics, such as the act of harvesting. In the New Testament, humanity is pictured as a field of ripening grain. Those who share the good news of Jesus are the workers who harvest men and women for God's kingdom (Matt. 9:37–38). The book of Revelation is recognized as having much symbolism representing the second coming of Christ (Rev. 1:12, 16, 20).

God's use of symbolism for me was surprising at first but reasonable since I tend to look for an underlying message or meaning. God knew that symbolism would create a dynamic mental picture for me, fostering greater understanding, translating into greater submission and acceptance. It worked. My dance with God was evidence of that. The use of symbolism began to occur so frequently that I started to look for it. One morning as I was eating breakfast, I suddenly realized what I was eating: Life cereal. Needless to say, this became my favorite breakfast food over the next several months as I symbolically ingested the fullness of "life" with every bite. "In Him is life, and the life is the light of men" (John 1:4).

Meditative Thought

In what ways, typical and atypical, has God reached out to you?

This lesson is dedicated to the memory of Daunte Barlow, a kind-hearted coworker and friend. Daunte displayed tremendous perseverance and patience throughout his battle with lupus, always with a smile on his face. God reached out to me through Daunte as we shared many laughs about our bald heads.

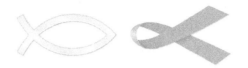

CLEAR MARGINS

Then your light will break out like the dawn, and your recovery will speedily spring forth.
—Isaiah 58:8

Clear margins—the term used to denote the line of demarcation where cancerous cells once were but are no more. In other words, normal cells are now present where a tumor once was. There are no sweeter words to a cancer patient and their loved ones than those two words. Two simple words, yet words packed with incomprehensible relief.

DECISIONS, DECISIONS

Surgery, when possible, may be necessary at the onset of a cancer diagnosis or it may be followed by other treatments such as chemotherapy. Each case is unique. Typically, the goal of cancer surgery is to attempt to achieve clear margins. Sometimes that is not possible, but this may not be known until the time of surgery. Sometimes a second surgery may even be required.

After my diagnosis, the surgeon informed Parker and me of the options available to us. We wanted to be fully informed before making our final decision, but in order to do that we needed to meet with a plastic surgeon. We wanted to explore the possibilities of reconstructive surgery following a mastectomy, should we decide to choose that route. Parker and I felt the most conservative surgical approach (lumpectomy) was our best option, but we had to be sure.

We visited the plastic surgeon's office and were led into a video room. Within minutes of watching a reconstructive procedure and listening to the detailed explanation, Parker and I found ourselves squirming and groaning. We looked at one another in shock and dismay. How were such things possible? It was remarkable, no doubt. We talked throughout the remainder of the video to cover the audio and calm our anxieties. The receptionist finally came in much to our relief to escort us into the next room.

The room was homey, decorated in soft colors accentuated by an overstuffed sofa with matching pillows. A long-stem flower arrangement sat in the corner. I am sure it was all intended to induce a sense of peace and tranquility. Try as it may, it had the opposite effect on me. I felt overcompensated and threatened. My discernment proved to be correct as I sensed we were in the wrong place. "This is what the Lord says: 'At just the right time, I will respond to you'" (Isa. 49:8 NLT).

Identify a time when God responded to you and you recognized it immediately (such as an answered prayer, avoidance of an accident, a greeting card with a meaningful message):

_____

_____

The plastic surgeon walked in, sat down, and proceeded to tell Parker and me why we only had one logical choice: a mastectomy. This was the best option. *Hmmm . . . did he mean for him or for me?* I wondered. He explained how my tissue would be forever damaged and we would have to endure the effects of radiation if I were to have a lumpectomy. However, if I had a mastectomy, I could forego the radiation altogether and have reconstructive surgery. *Some choice!* My skin would still be supple and natural-feeling as opposed to being dense and firm. *So what?* I silently retaliated. My blood pressure rose with each spoken word. How dare this stranger who just met us say there was only one right decision for us to make. Furthermore, how shallow to think my husband only loved me for my supple skin! I stood in anger when he began telling Parker what he would do if I were his wife, trying to appeal to Parker's sense of guilt. As we collected our belongings, the surgeon bellowed that we would be back to see him at some point. *Not in my lifetime,* I thought. In mid-sentence, Parker and I thanked him for his time and promptly walked out of the room. It was at that moment we made our final and firm decision: I would have a lumpectomy—unequivocally, undeniably, most assuredly, a lumpectomy. No more pondering the pros and cons. No more weighing the options. It was settled. The plastic surgeon had made certain of that. I immediately marched over to Dr. Winchester's office in the next building to inform her of my decision and schedule my surgery. I breathed a confident sigh of relief. At least that part was over. "Sustain me according to Thy word, that I may live; and do not let me be ashamed of my hope" (Ps. 119:116).

God provided double confirmation of our decision: the negative experience from the plastic surgeon's office and the positive feedback from my boss. Dr. Triozzi, an oncologist, agreed that the most conservative approach was just as effective as the most radical one, at least in my case. This may be a matter of medical debate, but it was good enough for me.

Describe a time when God provided confirmation of a decision for you.

_____

_____

_____

"ALL THE LOVE"

I was eager to have surgery and get the cancer out of my body. The day of my surgery came quickly. I stayed up late the night before, unable to sleep, feeling as if I had to complete my to-do list. It reminded me of how I get before going on vacation. Everything has to be in order (clothes washed and put away, dishwasher emptied, mail read, bills paid, etc.) But here I was busily writing last minute e-mails after midnight. We had to be at the hospital by 6 A.M., which meant I had to get up before 5 A.M. to curl my hair. I wanted my long, flowing hair to be perfect. Since I could not wear makeup, I would at least have great-looking hair. It just made me feel better. Maybe my visitors would focus on my hair and not on my pale face.

I was thrilled at the "standing room only" crowd in my hospital room. So many wonderful people came to wish me well. There was laughter, hugging, and hand-holding. Friends and family encircled Parker and me as they prayed for a successful surgery and subsequent recovery. When the escort came to take me to radiology for the needle localization procedure, she smiled and spoke of "all the love in that room." It gave me a feeling of warmth and gratitude knowing so many people cared about me and took the time to show it.

The needle localization procedure is a method used to identify the exact tumor location. It is not a pleasant experience. Though not mandatory, my surgeon opted for the procedure based upon my tumor characteristics. A thin hook wire tip is positioned at the tumor site to assist the surgeon. Most women are given valium to calm their nerves before having this procedure. I chose not to. *What was I thinking?* I wanted to be fully in the moment. *Again, what was I thinking?* Actually, I wanted to test my faith in relying on God to calm my fears. I did well until the radiologist left me alone in the room for an extended period of time. It was during that time that an unusual feeling came over me. I have felt like this only a few times before. It can best be described as if it felt like I would have an anxiety attack, crawl out of my skin, or scream like a raving lunatic down the hall if I allowed myself to succumb to my human nature. I entertained the idea of walking out of the hospital, foregoing the surgery, but there was a stronger spirit within me. It prevailed to fight off the fleshly inclinations, allowing God's peace to flow like a mighty river. I could tell it was not just in me but in the entire room. I relished the moment because I knew I was in God's presence, and His peace was there to overcome my anxiety. "For thus says the Lord, 'Behold, I extend peace to her like a river'" (Isa. 66:12).

Have you ever experienced God's peace taking precedence over your unsettling circumstances? Briefly explain.

_____

_____

During this moment of solitude, another interesting thing happened. God began to invade my mind with the thought of animals, correlating their characteristics to His attributes. In turn, His attributes were applied to my current situation. For example, an elephant symbolizes strength; God is stronger and more powerful than any force of nature, any mighty ocean, and certainly any disease. "Your faith should not rest on the wisdom of man, but on the power of God" (1 Cor. 2:5). The tiger symbolizes quiet ease of step and stalking of prey. God had placed the skills needed in my surgeon's hands to find the cancer and remove it. "Heal me, O Lord, and I will be healed; save me and I will be saved, for Thou art my praise" (Jer. 17:14). A lion is considered to be a fearless king or ruler in its domain. *Fearless, that's good.* "The wicked flee when no one is pursuing, but the righteous are bold as a lion" (Prov. 28:1). On and on my mind clicked from animal to animal, until the radiologist and his accomplice came back into the room. They couldn't believe I was still calm, especially with no valium. I knew why.

What kind of animal comes to your mind that might be indicative of your current situation? Relate God's attributes to this animal and how He can overcome.

_____

_____

The needle localization procedure was completed, and I was wheeled back into my room sporting a conspicuous urine container covering a protruding needle in my breast. I was glad my visitors were gone and only family remained, which was embarrassing enough. It wasn't long before the same escort returned to my room to take me to the surgery holding area. I asked to remain sitting straight up in bed so I could observe my surroundings. This seemed to be an unusual request. Most patients are sleeping or groggy at this point, but the escort and I enjoyed talking. She told me she'd never met anyone like me, asking how I was able to be so calm especially since this was my first surgery. I didn't hesitate to tell her and she was prompted to share her appreciation by giving me—get this—a small stuffed elephant with the hospital's logo! I laughed without explanation and thanked God for His humor and His presence. I still have the elephant, along with a lion given to me by the same escort who remembered me when I returned a few weeks later for a portacath implant.

ONE KNIFE UNDER GOD

I vaguely remember my arm being stretched out and strapped down. I heard someone comment that I was awake as Dr. Winchester entered the surgical suite. She said a short prayer and the surgery began. The surgery took longer than expected, partly because the lumpectomy required more tissue to be removed than was originally intended. In fact, it took two rounds to achieve clear margins. A "frozen section" confirmed the desired result. A frozen section is a piece of tissue that is snap-frozen and quick-stained, then viewed microscopically to see where (and if) the transition of abnormal cells to normal cells appears.

Another reason for the longer surgery was that the lymph node dissection was more invasive than anticipated. Dr. Winchester literally had to dig for the quarter-sized lymph node within the pit of my arm. It was so deep she was surprised I ever felt it. She was correct in one sense that I could only feel the node in certain awkward positions. However, I considered that to be just another of God's promptings to alert me to a more serious problem. Along with the "greatly enlarged grossly positive lymph node" as specified in the pathology report, Dr. Winchester also removed eight other normal-sized lymph nodes that proved to be negative.

As a matter of information the extent of the lymph node dissection is a discretionary decision by the surgeon at the time of surgery. The number of lymph nodes removed, if any, is limiting so as to minimize the compromised effect upon one's immune function. The lymphatic system serves as a source of circulation for cancerous cells, so this is a critical decision. There are some tests that may assist the surgeon's decision prior to surgery, but I did not undergo any of these.

My next recollection was one of pain—severe, intense pain—like "the way it must feel when you have been stabbed" kind of pain. I have never felt pain like that before and hope I never do again. I heard the nurse say I had not yet received any pain medication. Parker held my hand as tears rolled into my ears from the excruciating pain. I was taken to a private room where family and friends joined me. I was then informed of the good news for having clear margins and the bad news for possible aggressive chemotherapy due to the apparent malignant lymph node. This was devastating to me. I couldn't get the term *aggressive* out of my mind. What exactly did that mean? I knew up front I would have to go through radiation, but I had not planned to go through chemotherapy.

Dr. Winchester decided to admit me to the hospital overnight, but I didn't complain since morphine was only a nurses' call button away. Parker endured the restless night with me, returning from the house with a change of clothes and a dozen roses. I kept those roses and other flowers I received and allowed them to dry out. I then crumbled and put them in a glass keepsake jar. The potpourri of my flowers sits in a UAB Cancer Center jar in my curio cabinet alongside the dried crumbled flowers from my daddy's funeral a year earlier.

The next afternoon I was released to go home. It felt good to be in my own bed. My pain was manageable, but the drain tube protruding from my side was most uncomfortable. My recovery was speedy as we had prayed, but I did not regain full use of my arm for weeks. I became adept at doing twice as much with my other arm. I forced myself to be patient and forgiving with my progress. My dogs, however, were not so forgiving. They still wanted their afternoon walk!

Meditative Thought

What can God do specifically for you or your loved one if facing surgery?

This lesson is dedicated to Elizabeth Nunnelley, whom I fondly call Aunt Lib. She is a breast cancer survivor of many years and a tireless servant of God who enjoys ministering behind the scenes as she goes about touching the lives of many.

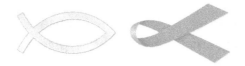

THE SHEPHERD'S COMFORT

The Lord is my shepherd, I shall not want.

—Psalm 23:1

In Isaiah 40, the prophet begins with a declaration of comfort to the people in captivity in Judah: "'Comfort, O comfort My people,' says your God" (Isa. 40:1). God comes with absolute power; but before the extent of God's almighty power is revealed, He is first described as a caring and compassionate shepherd. The Shepherd God is the context in which all His power is revealed. Isaiah wants us to understand the profound extent of God's might is seen in the way He shepherds His people.

AFFECTION FOR THE BLEATING

As stated earlier, my plan of action addressed not only a treatment plan but also a spiritual plan. I wanted—no, I needed—to connect with God in a way that brought me comfort and was a continuous reminder of His presence. This became most apparent with my first oncology visit. I craved comfort and reassurance in the midst of the structured chaos as I stood in line to schedule my next doctor's appointment along with what seemed like a flock of other oncology patients. I desperately needed strength and comfort when hopelessness and defeat were an easier option. How was I ever going to make it through this journey? How would I find comfort in the midst of each new crisis?

Wait a minute—a flock. I was part of the "flock" in the oncology clinic—like a flock of sheep. "My people have become lost sheep" (Jer. 50:6). *I was lost, all right.* My mind began to race. A sheep, I was like a sheep in a flock being herded through the gate as I stood there in line. "We are His people and the sheep of His pasture" (Ps. 100:3).

As I began to uncover my newly discovered analogy, I not only felt like a sheep, I wanted to be a sheep—a sheep in His pasture. Why? Because then I would have a shepherd to take care of me. "I am the good shepherd; and I know My own, and My own know Me" (John 10:14). God Almighty would be my shepherd, my very own personal shepherd; and I could rely on His protection at all times, day and night. "For thus says the Lord God, 'Behold, I Myself will search for My sheep and seek them out. As a shepherd cares for his herd in the days when he is among his scattered sheep, so I will care for My sheep and will deliver them from all the places to which they were scattered on a cloudy and gloomy day'" (Ezek. 34:11–12). The symbolism was uncanny as I considered the benefits of being a sheep, His sheep. My anxiety level dissipated with each new symbolic realization. Like a sheep, I needed tending. "'I myself will tend my sheep and cause them to lie down in peace,' says the Sovereign Lord" (Ezek. 34:15). I needed direction and guidance. "The sheep follow him because they know his voice" (John 10:4). I needed protection. "For you were continually straying like sheep, but now you have returned to the Shepherd and Guardian of your souls" (1 Pet. 2:25). But most of all, I needed comfort. "Thy rod and Thy staff, they comfort me" (Ps. 23:4). I was able to focus on my need for a shepherd as I relinquished my inadequacies to my Shepherd's incomparable ability.

Read or recite Psalm 23.
Does Psalm 23 bring you comfort? If so, how?

_____

_____

Yes, Lord, let me rest in green pastures; lead me beside still waters. Restore my health as we walk together through the valley of the shadow of death that cancer brings.

CASTING MY CARES

I have always heard how sheep are God's dumbest, most unenlightened creatures. Sheep are clueless when it comes to direction, and they will wander into dangerous territory looking for the next tasty nibble. It is in the valleys, though, where the richest green pastures are found—the most dangerous place in which to graze. The shepherd must lead the sheep to the mountaintop, away from danger. Not only are sheep directionless, they are defenseless. Their short, weak leg muscles, combined with bad eyesight and stubby horns, provide no defense against their predators. They are reliant on the shepherd to protect them.

Sometimes, in order to protect a continuously wandering sheep, the shepherd may have to break its leg for its own safety. This sounds harsh but then a sweet thing happens. Immediately afterwards, the shepherd will splint the leg and carry the sheep on his shoulders until the bone heals. Then, the sheep that had been so stubborn will be the sheep that stays the closest to the shepherd. I love that.

Sheep are fearful. A shepherd has to dam water to create a still pond before the sheep will drink from it because they are afraid of flowing water. When night falls, the sheep are called by name into the fold, each one counted and inspected by the shepherd for disease or wounds. If a healing agent is needed, the shepherd uses a mixture of oil, sulfur, and tar to apply to the suffering sheep. This not only provides comfort but also acts as an insecticide.

Here's my favorite sheep-like characteristic: when a sheep falls, causing it to roll over on its back, it becomes "cast." A cast sheep cannot right itself without the aid of the shepherd. It lies there helpless until rescued. If the sheep is not rescued, it will die due to trapped gases in its four stomachs which will cut off the circulation.[1] As a new cancer patient, I felt like a cast sheep, defenseless and totally dependent upon my Shepherd to rescue me. I felt this way many times, needing to be watched over and uprighted from my helpless, cast state.

Which of these sheep-like characteristics do you exhibit?

_____ dependent

_____ intelligence-deprived

_____ defenseless

_____ directionless

_____ continuously wandering

_____ fearful

_____ easily distracted

_____ cast

I think we can see ourselves with most, if not all, of these characteristics at one time or another. It was not long after my symbolic reassurance and newfound imagery that my friend, Sharon, gave me a small ceramic sheep. She had no idea of the contrived sheep analogy I was using to bring about spiritual comfort. She just saw a ceramic sheep when she was out and about one day and wanted me to have it. I took the figurine from her as tears began to well. It was a sheep lying on its back with all four feet in the air! I looked at it in disbelief. The sheep also had a content look on its face even though it was cast. What a precious gift, perfect in every way. I clutched the little sheep in my hands as if to remind me that although I was not able, my Shepherd was. Numerous times throughout the course of my treatments, I held tightly to that sheep needing the spiritual reassurance to nurture and sustain me. Even now when I want to feel God's closeness, I sometimes take that sheep and press its feet against my hand. I can almost hear the words, "Let me be your Shepherd today. I am able."

Describe a time when you felt like a cast sheep and the Shepherd rescued you.

_____

_____

_____

THE COMFORT OF HIS HOLINESS

Comfort comes in many forms: gentle words, a loving touch, an encouraging note, a cup of hot tea, soft music, or a furry companion. However, there is nothing more lasting, more encompassing, than the true source of comfort: the comforter Himself, the Holy Spirit. Let's consider for a moment who the Holy Spirit is and what He can provide. These verses give insight into the descriptive nature of the Holy Spirit. Identify the characteristic(s) in each verse.

Luke 12:12 _____

John 14:26 _____

Acts 1:8 _____

Acts 2:38 _____

Ephesians 1:3 _____

Isaiah 63:14_____

Romans 14:17_____

Romans 15:13_____

Titus 3:5_____

Power is revealed through the attributes of the Holy Spirit. We can see the nature and promise of the Holy Spirit through teaching, helping, renewing, righteousness, abiding within us, and providing peace, joy, hope, and rest. The Holy Spirit is a gift to all who believe. When we lean upon the grace and attributes of God the Father, Son, and Holy Spirit, we are reminded of His holiness and how it pervades every facet of His character. "There is no one holy like the Lord, indeed, there is no one besides Thee." (1 Sam. 2:2). It is within His holiness where we find focus, clarity, purpose, and on a more personal level, deep, abiding comfort. "So the church throughout all Judea and Galilee and Samaria enjoyed peace, being built up; and, going on in the fear of the Lord and in the comfort of the Holy Spirit, it continued to increase" (Acts 9:31).

Some refuse the comfort of the Holy Spirit. Rachel and Jacob refused comfort while mourning for their children (Gen. 37:35, Jer. 31:15). To experience comfort, we must accept it. Being receptive to the comfort His holiness can bring, gives us the reassurance we need to make it through our trials. "Thou, who hast shown me many troubles and distresses, wilt receive me again, and wilt bring me up again from the depths of the earth. Mayest Thou increase my greatness, and turn to comfort me" (Ps. 71:20–21).

Most of us, however strong we think we are, need to be reminded of the comfort we have available through the Holy Spirit. That is why I have produced a CD that musically depicts the "baby steps" needed to come into full recognition of the comfort only the Holy Spirit can bring. Each contemporary Christian song or instrumental arrangement reveals a step closer to the final step of giving thanks and offering a sacrifice of praise to God. (For information on how to obtain a copy of this CD, see the end of this lesson.)

In her booklet, *A Tea to Comfort Your Soul,* Emile Barnes said, "I think sometimes we miss out on the comfort and contentment God has for us because we insist on finding it where we want to find it—in the form that we want to find it—instead of opening our minds and our hearts to receive it as God wants to give it."[2] How about in the form of a sheep?

Meditative Thought

Let's bring it all together. How does being a sheep, comfort, the Holy Spirit, and contentment all relate to one another?

This lesson is dedicated to Elizabeth Fourie, an amazing Christian, encourager, comforter, and pastor's wife, who never lost sight of God's abiding presence throughout her cervical cancer. Her tireless efforts to the needs of others are beyond my understanding.

Note: The CD entitled *The Comfort of His Holiness* is a collection of seventeen contemporary Christian songs and instrumental arrangements meant to provide reassurance in times of personal crisis (not just cancer). Many of the songs reminded me of God's abiding presence as I endured my trials with cancer. For a $10 donation that includes shipping and handling, you may receive a copy. Please contact me at **karen@confrontingcancerwithfaith.com** to request your copy.

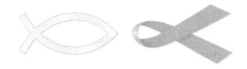

A BETTER PERSPECTIVE

Bring balm for her pain; perhaps she may be healed.

—Jeremiah 51:8

We all know it's better to see the glass half-full rather than half-empty. A positive perspective points us toward a positive attitude, resulting in a more positive outcome. Christian author and speaker Joyce Meyer says, "It's especially important to maintain a positive attitude because God is positive. And when we are positive, it releases Him to work in our lives."[3]

I am inspired by the story of a young man who lost his sight and became bitter and depressed. In an effort to help, a caring friend asked the blind man to create an extensive list of all the things he could still do. The list should include such things as still being able to smell flowers, feel the wetness of his dog's nose, hear the sound of his alarm clock, and so on. The blind man thought about it and began composing a list. It grew to be over a thousand things and was still growing the next time he saw his friend. Astonished at the list, the friend asked what made the difference in his radical new attitude. The answer: since he had decided to focus on all the things he could do, it drastically reduced his limitations of what he could not do. He had developed a better perspective.

THE SKINNY ON CHEMOTHERAPY VS. RADIATION THERAPY

As you will read several times throughout this study, a positive perspective and a God-centered attitude have a lot to do with acceptance and healing. Chemotherapy and/or radiation therapy often comprise a significant portion of one's cancer journey, offering plenty of opportunity and testing grounds for developing positive approaches. This lesson and the next will focus on chemotherapy and radiation therapy and how I incorporated a better perspective. Here's a good start: "Greater is He who is in you than he who is in the world" (1 John 4:4).

Let's first be clear about what chemotherapy and radiation therapy are. Chemotherapy is the treatment of cancer with drugs (chemicals) that destroy cancer cells. It is a systemic approach that attempts to accomplish one of three things depending on the cancer type and how advanced it is: cure the cancer, control the cancer, or relieve symptoms caused by the cancer. Some drugs work better together than alone, so two or more drugs are commonly given at the same time. There are also drugs that can be used to block the effect of the body's hormones or boost the immune system. This approach is known as "biological therapy." I have been involved with research in this area. Neither chemotherapy nor biological therapy is necessary for every cancer patient—your doctor will determine what is right for you or your loved one. Oftentimes chemotherapy is used in conjunction with surgery, radiation therapy, and/or biological therapy.[4]

When cancer invades the lymph nodes, like it did mine, a systemic approach of chemotherapy may be warranted. My one positive lymph node resulted in six cycles of aggressive chemotherapy over the course of eighteen weeks. Although standard and/or experimental chemotherapy is optional and there are other holistic alternatives, I would not have been satisfied following any plan other than my doctor's recommendations. Was it difficult? You bet! Did I get sick? Duh. Did I lose my hair? Yep, every stinking strand! Was the chemotherapy worth it? For me, absolutely.

Radiation therapy, in contrast to chemotherapy, is a localized approach that treats most solid tumors using penetrating beams of high-energy waves or streams of particles known as "radiation." Radiation therapy delivers specific amounts of radiation directly to the cancer site. Both chemotherapy and radiation therapy kill cancer cells, but the down side is that they also kill healthy cells (which usually repair themselves following treatment). The harm to healthy cells is what causes side effects. It is important to understand that these side effects, whether severe or minimal, are not an indicator of treatment effectiveness, as this varies significantly from person to person.[5]

Do you or your loved one have fears or unanswered questions about chemotherapy and/or radiation therapy? If so, write them down and discuss them with a medical professional.

PULSATING POISON VS. HEALING BALM

Now that I have discussed the primary differences between chemotherapy and radiation therapy, let's get personal. How did I endure it? What were some of my coping tactics? How did I develop a better perspective?

During my second treatment I came to realize how important it was to view chemotherapy in a positive light. I decided to stop referring to it as "poison" and instead refer to it as a "healing balm"—hence, the focal verse for today. I extended my positive thinking into my daily conversation. I told my close friends I did not want to hear anything—and I meant anything—negative. Only positive input was allowed. Wanting to help, my friend Sharon wrote uplifting Bible verses on index cards, laminated them, and instructed me to place them in strategic locations throughout my house (bathroom mirror, wig stand, prescription box). Each card served as an encouragement that troubled times would pass and God was with me. "My soul waits in silence for God only, for my hope is from Him. He only is my rock and my salvation, my stronghold; I shall not be shaken" (Ps. 62:5–6).

Write two comforting Bible verses on an index card and place them in a frequented location. Which verses did you choose and where do you plan to place them?

_____

_____

One thing I did to stay upbeat during the chemotherapy was to reward myself. Prior to each treatment, I bought a new CD. I made the shopping excursion something to anticipate, which helped to distract my focus from the chemo and its unpleasant side effects. While I admit I didn't always listen to the CD during my treatment as planned, I still purchased one. The plan worked well until my fifth treatment. For some reason, my fifth treatment was one of distinct dread. The cumulative side effects were hard to ignore, but the nausea was finally under control having tried three different medications. I had been told the hardest part of chemo was getting adjusted to the chemo dosage and finding the proper medicine to control the side effects. Ditto to that. However, once that was regulated, it was tolerable.

What is one way for you to maintain a positive perspective in the midst of a negative situation (not necessarily chemo)?

_____

_____

One simple thing that helped my husband cope with all of this chemotherapy "stuff" was to include him in the first treatment. Parker is not comfortable with hospitals, needles, doctors, and the like; but he came to infusion therapy with me to see what was involved. He helped me settle into a comfortable easy chair while Kendra, my nurse, introduced herself and explained what was about to happen. She proceeded to access the portacath in my shoulder to administer the chemotherapy. Parker cringed. She administered three separate agents: one looked like a large syringe of bright red Kool-Aid® while the other two were clear in color. Each was given slow and deliberately. Parker watched with a wary eye until he was satisfied I was in good hands. After that day, Parker either waited in the lobby or dropped me off and came back to pick me up.

Mistakes Made, Insights Gained

In retrospect, I recall some mistakes I made throughout the course of my chemotherapy. One was the deception of what I would be able to do following a treatment. Because I felt OK immediately following my first treatment—in fact, much better than anticipated—Parker and I decided to go to a local seafood restaurant for lunch. I ordered a pasta shrimp dish with creamy white sauce. I had been warned that was not the best idea, but I didn't see what all the fuss was about. Following the meal, Parker and I decided to go to a movie to get our mind off the day's events. Halfway through the movie, "it" hit me. I mean, "it" hit me like a ton of bricks. My body felt like lead was being poured into it, the nausea started kicking in, my head got fuzzy, and the "ick factor" began to escalate. We left in the nick of time. My take-home lesson from that experience was that side effects are not always immediate. I also learned the importance of taking all of my medications exactly as directed. We discovered after-the-fact I had gotten off-track with one of the medications. After that, Parker made a computer spreadsheet of my medication schedule.

Another mistake I made was not to rest when I felt the need. I pushed myself at times when it might have been wiser to stay home. I was very fortunate to have a job that was flexible and a boss who was supportive. My job was the last thing for which I needed to be concerned. This was a tremendous blessing. I had chosen to continue working so I could maintain a semblance of normalcy. I realize that is not a viable option for everyone. Insurance, finances, job demands, and unsupportive personnel can present major problems. Work issues are often a major area of concern for patients and their caregivers. If this is true for you, this is just one more area to lift up to the Lord and watch Him work. Here are some verses that might be helpful:

- Lift up your eyes—"For my eyes are toward Thee, O God, the Lord; in Thee I take refuge; do not leave me defenseless" (Ps. 141:8).
- Thank Him in advance for what He will do—"He rescued me, because He delighted in me" (Ps. 18:19).
- Believe it, live it—"I will put my trust in Him" (Heb. 2:13).

Here a few verses I read on my first day of chemotherapy:

- "The Lord is good, a stronghold in the day of trouble, and He knows those who take refuge in Him" (Nah. 1:7).
- "Be strong and courageous! Do not tremble or be dismayed, for the Lord your God is with you wherever you go" (Josh. 1:9).

Find a Bible verse that speaks encouragement and hope to you. Write it below and memorize it.

_____

_____

GOD'S PERSPECTIVE: THE BEST PERSPECTIVE

In 2004 a catastrophic tsunami hit Asia, killing thousands of people and leaving others homeless, jobless, penniless, and/or orphaned. Many responded to the vast recovery efforts. Posters of the missing were displayed everywhere, bodies lined the streets, mass graves were dug; the stench of death was all around. A debate erupted as to what God's role and/or intent in this horrific event might have been. One commentator posed the question, "Will we see God in the angry ocean rising up to destroy all life in its wake, or will we see God in the care of millions of strangers rising up to save life and care for the human hurts?" It's not a matter of understanding but rather a matter of perspective and faith. We can't answer hard questions; but we can, and must, accept that God is good all the time. "Why are you asking Me about what is good? There is only One who is good" (Matt. 19:17). Maintaining a godly perspective is one of the most powerful ways to acknowledge that God is greater than our circumstances.

Look at the twelve men Moses sent out as spies into the land of Canaan. All twelve had inspected the same territory, yet ten came back with a negative report and two—Joshua and Caleb—had a positive report. The ten said, "We are not able to go up against the people for they are too strong for us" (Num. 13:31). But the two said, "We should by all means go up and take possession of it, for we shall surely overcome it" (Num. 13:30). Who would you believe? It depends on your perspective and faith, doesn't it?

Who proved to be correct in possessing the land—the ten or the two? _____ (Numbers 15:2)

Joseph, the favored son of Jacob, is another example. Joseph demonstrated a positive perspective in spite of being sold into slavery by his jealous brothers, in spite of being thrown into prison for being falsely accused of attempted rape of his master's wife, in spite of having interpreted the dreams of two of the king's officials who promised to remember him upon their prison release but never made good on their promise, and in spite of having lived apart from his family and homeland for many years. Joseph never lost a godly perspective. He told his brothers, "You meant evil against me, but God meant it for good in order to bring about this present result" (Gen. 50:20). Wherever he was, whatever he did, God made Joseph to prosper. In the depths of a pit, while in prison, in the king's court, and while serving as overseer of Egypt during times of severe drought, it didn't matter: Joseph carried God in his heart.

There is a lesson to be learned from Joshua, Caleb, and Joseph. The lesson is that you can have a godly perspective in spite of difficult circumstances.

Becky Sue Fitch, an alumnus from my alma mater of the University of Southern Mississippi said, "On most days I like to think of myself as living with cancer rather than dying from it."[6] She has surely learned the value of a positive perspective.

Meditative Thought

Hands

A basketball in my hands is worth about $19.
A basketball in Michael Jordan's hands is worth about $33 million.

A slingshot in my hands is a kid's toy.
A slingshot in David's hand is a mighty weapon.

A rod in my hands will keep away an angry dog.
A rod in Moses' hand will part the mighty sea.

Two fish and five loaves of bread in my hands are a couple of fish sandwiches.
Two fish and five loaves of bread in Jesus' hand will feed thousands.

Nails in my hands might produce a birdhouse.
Nails in Jesus' hand will produce salvation for the entire world.

—Author unknown

This lesson is dedicated to my faithful canine companions—Frezno, Skippy, Alamo, and Susie—who showed unconditional love, devotion, and comfort throughout my chemotherapy. Their constantly happy disposition with life reminded me that a better perspective goes a long way.

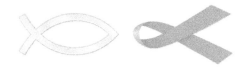

"X" MARKS THE SPOT

Strength and dignity are her clothing, and she smiles at the future.
—Proverbs 31:25

An "X" on a map indicates a final destination; an "X" on a test selects a chosen answer; an "X" on an application form indicates the signature line; and an "X" on a letter symbolizes a kiss. However, an "X" in radiation therapy has a whole different meaning. The X's are temporary "tattoos." I admit it is better than the "artwork" of yesteryear when patients were painted with unsightly black patterned outlines anywhere and everywhere on their body. I had dreaded this "body mapping" for months knowing, but not realizing to the extent, how humiliating it would be. Black X's were colored all over my half-naked body as if I had become a connect-a-dot game board. And if that wasn't embarrassing enough, snapshots had to be taken!

The X's, though degrading, served a vital purpose. They marked the location where the radiation would be strategically applied to exactness day after day throughout treatments. This was important so that the radiation did not incorporate any more healthy cells than was absolutely necessary. Mapping is all part of the simulation procedure providing information for complex calculations that determine the best possible delivery of radiation specific to your body structure. For me, the radiation plan to deliver sixty-five gys (pronounced "grays," formally referred to as "rads") over the course of thirty-six treatments (about seven weeks), would involve a small segment of my heart and the uppermost tip of my lung. While it bothered me, it was unavoidable.

MARKED BY GOD

As I considered the necessity of being marked by the radiation team, I compared it to being marked as a child of God. The symbolism seemed much more palatable. I thought about when the Israelites marked themselves as God's chosen on the night of the Lord's Passover. They were instructed to place the blood of an unblemished lamb on the doorposts of their houses. "And the blood shall be a sign for you on the houses where you live; and when I see the blood I will pass over you, and no plague will befall you to destroy you when I strike the land of Egypt" (Ex. 12:13).

I also thought about Paul. He had visible marks of persecution for the cause of Christ. "For I bear on my body the brand-marks of Jesus" (Gal. 6:17). And Christ Himself bore the marks of suffering that gave us eternal life. "'We have seen the Lord!' But he [Thomas] said to them, 'Unless I shall see in His hands the imprint of the nails, and put my finger into the place of the nails, and put my hand into His side, I will not believe'" (John 20:25).

As Christians, we are marked in the very heavens. "Rejoice that your names are recorded in heaven" (Luke 10:20). Even before the foundation of the world our names have been entered into the Lamb's book of life if you are a believer (Rev. 13:8). In addition we have a dwelling place reserved for us in heaven. "In My Father's house are many dwelling places; if it were not so, I would have told you; for I go to prepare a place for you" (John 14:2). It was easy for me to see how bearing the marks of Christ had their definite benefits.

As a believer, how are some ways that your life is personally "marked" by Christ?

_____

_____

If you are not a believer, then you do not carry the marks of Christ—but you can change that. If you are a believer, others should recognize it through your speech, actions, morals, and character.

THE WAITING ROOM

Several people told me that radiation therapy would be a breeze compared to chemotherapy. Then why did I feel so distraught? Why couldn't I convince myself that the radiation was more tolerable than the chemo? I began to analyze my uneasiness. The necessity of the radiation treatments had been made clear to me from the start. The treatments themselves lasted less than five minutes and no, they didn't hurt. But, it was those few minutes every day that caused me to rearrange my entire schedule over the course of the next two months. It was a constant reminder that I had cancer and there was no way I was going to forget it. I could not get any mental relief from its monotonous daily presence. At least with chemotherapy, my treatments were spaced out every three weeks.

The radiation oncology waiting room became a place of mental suffering for me, at least at first. As I sat there, refusing to watch television or engage in conversation, I found myself becoming anxious, especially when there was a delay. It was a real challenge for me to accept the idea I was diligently pursuing something I didn't even want to but, of course, needed to.

Have you ever pursued something you didn't want to but knew it was in your best interest? Explain.

_____

_____

After a week of self-induced anguish, I decided my waiting time would better be served redirecting my thoughts. I decided to bring devotional material to read—nothing too deep or thought-provoking, just something positive that included God in my morning waiting ritual. As I pursued this new approach, I began to sense an improved tolerance toward the cantankerous red laser radiation instrument known as a linear accelerator that was frequently in need of repair.

Many cancer patients and/or family members develop friendships, some of them lifelong, as they come to the common meeting grounds of the patient waiting room. I met one such woman about three weeks into my treatments. I was resistant to introduce myself at first, preferring to remain quiet and isolated as I read. But this woman intrigued me. She arrived early each morning, well before her scheduled appointment, with a nun dressed in her habit. The two often conversed with a younger woman being treated for a brain tumor. One day as we sat facing one another in the secondary waiting area, the older woman spoke to me. I responded, still not wanting to feel compelled to develop a casual friendship. Slowly, however, a bud of friendship began to sprout. I learned she was from Russia. She told me how God had preserved her and her husband as they endured the tremendous hardships of the Russian regime years ago. She beamed with joy as she spoke in her thick Russian brogue. I was fascinated. She encouraged me day after day with stories of God's love. God had sent her my way to lift my heavy spirit. She entered my life for that short season having served a noble purpose, and then she was gone. I never saw her again after I slipped a small gift into her hand on my last day of treatment.

Have you ever met someone for a season you felt God had sent your way? Explain.

_____

_____

HUMILIATION AND HUMILITY

As the two months of radiation progressed, it became harder and harder to find suitable clothes to wear that not only hid the telltale X's on my body but, more importantly, were comfortable. I was thankful for the local store specializing in cancer patients' needs equipping me with all the things to make my life more pleasant during this time including comfortable undergarments. The radiation had caused my skin to become red and sensitive, like an obsessed fair-skin sunbather. *What dummy would keep going out in the sun day after day after being sunburned?* I thought. Then I realized that at one point in my life, I was one of those dummies! I smiled.

I soon discovered that the X's were not limited to my body but were all over my clothes. For almost a year after treatments, I stumbled across an X on a bathing suit or pair of pajamas.

It was easy to be reminded of my humiliation whenever I stepped into the shower or changed clothes, because the black X's served to highlight my invisible blemishes. I became indignant with minimizing the marks placed upon me by those "cold and heartless techs" who were simply doing their job. If I had to have marks, at least they didn't have to be smeared. I used an alcohol pad to make sure the X's had a defined margin. For some reason, this gave me a feeling of satisfaction. If I were honest, maybe it was more an attempt of control. However, toward the end of my treatments, I found myself actually reinforcing the mark with my own Sharpie pen. It was as if I had stopped resisting and began conforming, having mentally accepted the underlying purpose and importance in my healing. "Clothe yourselves with humility toward one another, for God is opposed to the proud, but gives grace to the humble" (1 Pet. 5:5).

How can we properly clothe ourselves according to the verse in 1 Peter?

_____

An Unlikely Place of Worship

For two months, almost every morning I would lay half-naked on a cold table with my arm saddled flat over my head in an uncomfortable sling-like apparatus. I felt like a bulls-eye target as the red lasers danced over my chest for proper alignment. I rarely watched this procedure, either closing my eyes or looking straight up at the ceiling plastered with peace-inducing pictures. Once the alignment was complete, the radiation techs walked out of the room, shutting a thick, metal door behind them. I wondered if that was what a prison door sounded like. Soon I could hear a loud hum along with a whirring noise as the instrument positioned itself. Sometimes it sounded like a bouncing basketball.

I came to despise the humming sound. It made me feel like a hot dog in a microwave. I had to find some relief. At first I tried praying, hard, to refocus my attention and to try to drown out the noise. Then I tried singing praise songs in my mind to the key of "hmmmm." The faster the song, the better. I even opened my hands from my mummy-like position to offer praise to God. "For I am the Lord your God, who upholds your right hand, who says to you, 'Do not fear, I will help you'" (Isa. 41:13). A few times I sensed the presence of angels in the room. After awhile, my radiation therapy routine became a time of worship—a time, although I felt conformed to the demands of medical science, when I could reach out to grasp the waiting hand of my heavenly Father. "Ascribe to the Lord the glory due His name; bring an offering, and come before Him; worship the Lord in holy array" (1 Chron. 16:29). Once again, peace pervaded, allowing me to endure treatment after treatment until all thirty-six of them were over. Oh, happy day.

Do you have a song you like to offer God in times of stress? If not, think of one.

During my radiation therapy, my sweet husband, made me a treatment countdown calendar. I felt like a child counting down the days till Christmas. I placed the calendar on the refrigerator door and marked it with a pink X every day when I got home from work. Those were two of the longest months of my life. Needless to say, the X's on the calendar were much more satisfying than the ones on my body.

Meditative Thought

Have you found some unlikely places of worship? If so, where?

This lesson is dedicated to the memory of Jack Cox, Sr., who fearlessly served God and his country before succumbing to melanoma. He was such a man of joy with the mark of Christ on his life as seen through his contagious disposition.

Week 4

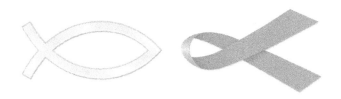

THE PROCESS: THE EFFECTS

The effects of cancer can be devastating to patients, family, and friends. Although the effects are not always pleasant—such as loss of hair, interruptions in your daily living, inconvenient appointments, or a continuum of setbacks—we can be molded into a stronger person. No doubt cancer has affected your relationships. Has the effect been good or bad? What about when you are faced with a poor prognosis? How do you effectively cope? Where do you find the encouragement, comfort, and hope you so desperately need? We can learn to accept the changes cancer brings through maturing our faith and walking with God each step of the way.

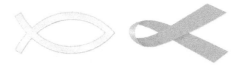

ACCEPTING CHANGE

God sees not as man sees, for man looks at the outward appearance,
but the Lord looks at the heart.

—1 Samuel 16:7

From the day you are diagnosed you will be forever changed," says cancer survivor, Susan Cambria. "This event will be added to the list of 'Where were you when . . .' Life becomes divided into B.C. (before cancer) and A.D. (after diagnosis). Believe it or not, you will come to celebrate perhaps the worst day of your life. It will become the yearly finish line in a never-ending race to outlive your disease. Birthdays will be celebrations of surviving another year instead of being dreaded reminders of aging. Accept that you will come through this journey a different person. You will get to know your true self and chances are you'll like yourself a lot more."[1] Amen, Sister Susan.

ACCEPTING OUR EXCEPTIONS

In the Lifetime movie, *Why I Wore Lipstick to My Mastectomy*, the cancer survivor boldly proclaims, "I am not my hair. I am not my skin." Let me add to that: "I am not a body part or a specimen." I am none of these things; but I am accepted, accepted by Christ. I am secure, I am loved; and I am significant. The things I am in Christ are the things that matter. They are things with eternal relevance. "There is, therefore, now no condemnation for those who are in Christ Jesus" (Rom. 8:1).

What is something you are not? I am not _____.

What is something you are in Christ? I am _____.

Knowing who we are in Christ gives us a stabilizing force when change blows into our lives. We can cling to the great I Am because He does not change. He is perfect. He is complete. There is nothing to be added or taken away. There is no change to be made to correct some flaw. "For I, the Lord, do not change" (Mal. 3:6). All that He touches is perfect: the rising and setting of the sun, the distribution of its heat, the crashing of the ocean waves, the placement of the stars—I could go on. "The law of the Lord is perfect, restoring the soul" (Ps. 19:7). We, on the other hand, are not perfect. We change. Our circumstances change, our jobs change, our health changes.

CHANGE, CHANGE GO AWAY

When change comes into our lives, we do one of three things: deny it, resist it, or accept it. Usually the last thing we do, or at least want to do, is accept it. While change itself can be difficult, accepting it can be even harder. And just because you accept something, does not mean you have to like it.

Why is acceptance important? For one thing, it promotes healing. It also allows you to live more at peace with yourself and with those around you. "Accept one another, just as Christ also accepted us to the glory of God" (Rom. 15:7). Accepting the changes in your life allow you to have a more positive outlook. This creates a more favorable environment to motivate, strengthen, and empower.

> When change comes into our lives, we do one of three things: deny it, resist it, or accept it.

Second, acceptance is an act of trust. In essence, you are saying, "God, I trust you to do with my life as you see fit. I don't understand all that is happening to me; but I relinquish my inadequacies, my fears, my heartaches, my life into Your capable hands." "And my God shall supply all your needs according to His riches in glory in Christ Jesus" (Phil. 4:19).

Third, acceptance propels you forward, ridding you of things that may hold you back. By accepting, you are better able to look ahead to the things that are yet to be. The act of acceptance filters out what you cannot change so you can walk with grace and honor. No woman should have to accept being bald or losing a breast, an ovary, or any other organ. No man should have to accept losing his hair either or his prostate. But if our health dictates otherwise, the sufficiency of God can pull us through. "I will instruct you and teach you in the way which you should go; I will counsel you with My eye upon you" (Ps. 32:8). So what are some practical ways to achieve acceptance? Let me share some pathways that have worked for me.

PATHWAYS TOWARD THE ROAD TO ACCEPTANCE

Rationalization. When I was eleven years old, my family moved from our modest house into a bigger house across town. It was exciting but it presented a dilemma: the house was located in a new school district. Living in this new district, I would have to forego the honor of becoming a school safety patrol. For years I had looked forward to being a safety patrol at Main Avenue Elementary School. After all, I had earned the privilege with my good grades. I would finally have the opportunity to flaunt my white safety belt for the world to see. I dreamed of helping students cross the street with my crisp, yellow safety flag. But now I would be attending Pinecrest Elementary. They didn't have safety patrols with white belts and yellow flags. I was heartbroken. How could I accept this awful change brought into my life? I rationalized that our new split-level house with its attic fan, two patios, and downstairs family room, not to mention the freshly painted big girls' blue bedroom and walk-in closet, was worth the sacrifice. My rationalization worked.

Displacement. Shortly after Parker and I were married, I snagged my first job as a medical technologist. Three months later Parker was notified of a transfer to southwest Louisiana. "That's Cajun country," I balked. "They eat nasty crawfish and talk funny." Besides, both of our families lived in

Alabama. How would I survive as a newlywed moving to another state? I dreaded the thought of finding another job and moving so far away, but solace soon came in the form of a mangy puppy. Parker allowed me to keep the stray pup I had picked up on the highway. Rosco brought immediate joy and comfort. With my new, ugly puppy, I could accept our new home, a new job, and a new culture. Rosceaux (our Cajun adaptation) displaced my sadness with joyful acceptance. Rosceaux eventually grew a full coat of fur and turned out to be a beautiful dog. As for the nasty mudbugs, there's nothing like 'em! I eat them every chance I get.

Renewal. The most challenging change in my life came with my cancer diagnosis. It deepened my faith, expanded my spirituality, and strengthened my character. It put into action the hope I have always had in Jesus Christ but prompted a renewal of His presence and fresh outpouring of His spirit. While I lamented the fact I had cancer, I knew deep in my heart the journey could bring me to a place of spiritual renewal, which it did. "In the way of righteousness is life, and in its pathway there is no death" (Prov. 12:28).

Reward. I'm all about rewards as incentives. Earlier I described the purchase of a new CD for each of my chemotherapy visits. Another example would be when my daddy would take the family to Florida to see my grandmother. I enjoyed visiting her and going to the beach, but I detested the drive that it took to get there. As a child, it seemed forever long. I knew there was nothing that could shorten the distance, so I focused on the doughnut and root beer stops I knew my daddy would make. If we were lucky, he might even make a boiled peanut stop. The trip was still long, but it helped to have rewards along the way.

Other pathways to acceptance include restoring, reclaiming, revitalizing, and repositioning. Have any of these pathways helped you achieve acceptance toward your or your loved one's cancer? If so, which one(s) and how?

_____

_____

I believe there is a three-step process that must happen to ensure adequate and complete acceptance for any chosen pathway. The three steps are: conformity, cooperation, and consolation—in that order. Conformity means to comply, to develop a harmonious agreement with cancer, so to speak, that moves beyond shock and denial. Cooperation is affiliated with action, in contrast to conformity, which is more like a state of mind. With both the mind and body in synchronization, consolation can be reached. Without all three steps, it is unlikely that acceptance can be fully achieved. In other words, it would be difficult to have cooperation without conformity, or consolation without cooperation. Once the last step of consolation has been achieved, you are ready to embrace life again.

An important concept I learned in achieving full acceptance was to do it in small increments. When I confessed to Parker that I was having difficulty grasping all the things cancer brought into my life, he suggested I focus on one day at a time. That was simple. Why hadn't I thought of that? It seemed so enlightening. One day at a time, one hour at a time, one moment at a time. Forget about next week. Stay in the moment. That one thing helped me tremendously. How you find acceptance is not as important as the fact that you do. God will help you through each step of the way. "And your ears will hear a word behind you, 'This is the way, walk in it,' whenever you turn to the right or to the left" (Isa. 30:21).

Loved ones as well as cancer patients need to reach a level of acceptance as to how cancer has affected their lives. Where are you in this process? Circle all that apply.

Conformity   Cooperation   Consolation   I am not ready to accept what is happening.

CHANGES IN THE CANCER PATIENT

Let's look through the lens of the cancer patient. First, understanding the disease helps facilitate accepting the changes it brings. So let me digress to address some basic facts. Although there are known risk factors and test predictors of cancer, no one can say if or when cancer will occur and/or how it will progress. What is known is that cancer is a group of more than a hundred different diseases. Normally the body's cells work cooperatively with the body's natural hormones, diet, and environment; but when the body's cells become abnormal for any reason and begin dividing out of control, gene alterations occur. A tumor can form, either benign or malignant. Malignant tumors invade, damage, and destroy nearby tissue and can spread to other parts of the body. A benign tumor won't spread, but it has the ability to still damage local tissue. Cancer cells from a malignant tumor can break away and enter the bloodstream and possibly the lymphatic system. This is how cancer spreads. That which has spread to other parts of the body is the same disease and has the same name as the original cancer but is called "metastatic." For example, breast cancer that has spread to the bones is called metastatic breast cancer, not bone cancer.[2]

Cancer can bring with it a host of unpleasant side effects such as: fatigue, nausea, vomiting, diarrhea, constipation, dietary challenges, skin irritation, hair loss, sore muscles, sore throat, sleeplessness, nail deterioration, mouth ulcers, difficulty swallowing, dry cough, induced menopause, susceptibility to infection, cognitive dysfunction, blurred vision, burning eyes, weight changes, tissue changes, swelling, anxiety, and depression. These side effects vary in degree and are as unique as the individual, the type of cancer, and the treatment.

Chemically-induced menopause was a difficult side effect for me. It commonly occurs in premenopausal women undergoing chemotherapy. I was greatly bothered by the uncomfortable symptoms of sudden menopause, but once I was able to identify them as symptoms of menopause and not chemotherapy per se, I was able to accept them with less anxiety. In fact, I was actually thankful for an explanation. Fortunately, my symptoms diminished post-chemotherapy—but that is not always the case.

What are some changes that you or your loved one has encountered since being diagnosed with cancer?

_____

_____

_____

CHANGED FOR GODLY GOOD

Daniel, Job, and Paul all recognized that change was from God. Daniel said, "Let the name of God be blessed forever and ever, for wisdom and power belong to Him. And it is He who changes the times and the epochs" (Dan. 2:20–21). Paul looked forward to change as he spoke about what would happen to the dead upon Christ's return. "Behold, I tell you a mystery; we shall not all sleep, but we shall all be changed, in a moment, the twinkling of an eye, at the last trumpet; for the trumpet will sound, and the dead will be raised imperishable, and we shall be changed" (1 Cor. 15:51–52). Notice Paul said twice that we would be changed. Job, the epitome of physical suffering and perseverance, demonstrated a down-to-earth viewpoint when he said, "Shall we indeed accept good from God and not accept adversity?" (Job 2:10) Good question. Shall we not accept the changes in our lives, still realizing God is in control? Short-term changes, long-term changes, lifetime changes—God is there. He has always been there. He always will be.

Meditative Thought

Is there a change in your life right now that you have been unable to accept? Ask God to change your heart.

This lesson is dedicated to my sweet friend and mentor Mary Nell Spraberry, a two-time cancer survivor. Her godly wisdom, study of the Word, and great anticipation of the Lord's return is to be admired. Mary Nell has learned to accept the changes life brings by trusting in the One who meets all her needs and directs her every path.

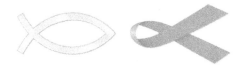

YOU'RE STILL BEAUTIFUL

He has made everything beautiful in its time.
—Ecclesiastes 3:11 NIV

Beauty is in the eye of the beholder." Isn't that what you hear when someone or something is essentially unattractive? Each morning when I looked in the mirror, I wondered how God could view me as beautiful. I certainly didn't look or feel beautiful with my twelve eyelashes and sixteen eyebrows. Yet because I believed God's Word, I knew I was. Many mornings I wrestled with human emotions versus godly truth in front of my bathroom mirror. I convinced myself day after day that even if no one else saw me as beautiful, God did; and that would have to be enough. "And let not your adornment be merely external—braiding the hair, and wearing gold jewelry, or putting on dresses; but let it be the hidden person of the heart, with the imperishable quality of a gentle and quiet spirit, which is precious in the sight of God" (1 Pet. 3:3–4).

A highlight of each day was getting the mail to see if any cards or notes of encouragement had come. (I think my mother had put the word out how much I loved to get mail.) One day I received a "praying for you" postcard sent from my church. It only had a line or two for a personal message. I had received many of these postcards, but I'll never forget the three handwritten words at the bottom of this particular one: "You are beautiful." I broke into tears. The sender didn't know I was almost bald and felt anything but beautiful. Reassurance and comfort flushed through me like a mild hot flash. I wish I could remember who wrote those words, but it was the perfect message at the perfect time. I thanked God.

No Hair Must Equal Cancer

There are many personal insults accompanying cancer. Some of them are visible, some are not. It is the visible ones that draw attention much like a flashing neon sign reading "I have cancer, I have cancer." No hair and, let's be honest, no breasts (much less one) are not natural for a woman. Society will allow a man to have a bald head and nobody gives a second look, but a female sporting a hairless noggin' becomes the eighth wonder of the world! Being bald was every bit as difficult for me as having cancer—at times, even harder. I hesitate to say it but it was true. Not every cancer patient feels that way but I sure did. Before having cancer, I never realized how significant and important my hair was to me or how much of my identity I placed on it. I had a full head of thick, long brown hair and had styled it in soft curls most of my life. In fact, I was so conditioned to having long hair that when I became bald and for months afterward, I still attempted to flip my hair out from under the collar of my shirt or jacket.

Hair began falling out and changing all over my body after my second chemo treatment. Even the hairs on my arms looked as if they had been singed. It was degrading, humiliating, and uncomfortable. It left me feeling exposed. Not only did I have cancer, now I had no hair, giving claim to the assumption "no hair equals cancer." But "no hair" did not have to equal "no beauty." "For God sees not as man sees, for man looks at the outward appearance, but the Lord looks at the heart" (1 Sam. 16:7).

What are some things God sees when He looks at your heart?

_____

_____

ENCOURAGE YOURSELF

I had been warned that the chemo would cause me to lose my hair, but I hoped against hope I would be an exception. I struggled over my imminent hair loss, knowing it would eventually grow back, but that did not bring me comfort. I didn't care about later. I cared about now. I despised the repeated reminders of, "It'll grow back." But you know what? They were right.

I considered writing myself a letter of encouragement early in the chemo so I could read it after all my hair was gone. That way I could be reminded in my own handwriting that this was temporary, and I was still beautiful to the most important person in my life: Jesus Christ. David, a man after God's own heart, often encouraged himself in the Lord. "In the day when I called thou answeredst me; thou didst encourage me with strength in my soul" (Ps. 138:3 ASV). On one occasion, David and his soldiers were distressed over the captivity of their wives and children by the Amalekites, who intended to make them slaves. With the people embittered and ready to stone David, he turned to God and encouraged himself in the Lord. Soon afterward, he overthrew the Amalekites and recovered all that had been taken (1 Sam. 30:1–18).

What is your first reaction when you feel defeated? What do you do or can you do to encourage yourself?

_____

_____

THE WIGFEST: A HAIR-OWING EXPERIENCE

I became suspicious the time was drawing near to lose my hair when my scalp began tingling. Every hair follicle on my head was sore—as if I had taken my hair down from an all-day high ponytail. A gentle head massage never felt better. An extra moisturizing shampoo specially formulated for chemotherapy-radiation hair loss helped some. No one gave me warning of an expected timeline. I didn't know if I would go bald all at once or if it would be extended over a period of time. (It actually occurred over a few weeks.) Nonetheless, I needed to come up with a plan and I needed it fast.

I had thought about using my own hair to fabricate a wig, but it would have required my hair to be cut to one-inch from my head. I wasn't ready for that. Plus the expense was extravagant, although Parker was agreeable. The advantages of having a wig with my own hair were obvious, the best one being it would allow me to continue styling it as I always had. You can't do that with a synthetic wig. Torn between what to do, I asked Parker to help me decide. All things considered, I chose to go with a synthetic wig. I called my friend Susan. She volunteered to go with me to a wig shop that catered to cancer patients. Susan was my angel making the trauma more bearable with her spirited personality and honest opinions. "Indeed, the very hairs of your head are all numbered. Do not fear; you are of more value than many sparrows" (Luke 12:7).

My criterion was simple: find the shortest-cut wig in my hair color. I must have tried on half the wigs in the store looking for the perfect one. I had not anticipated the difficulty in matching hair color to wig color, especially when the hair had various shades like mine did. I didn't want different hair colors or funky styles, just a conservative and professional-looking cut with which I could be comfortable. Finally, we found it—a short brown wig with sheer netting allowing for a natural-looking part. My sister Nancy teased me, suggesting I should use some white liquid paper to color in a few gray strands for a more realistic look!

My strategy was well-planned: find a wig, cut my hair to match it, and then take off the wig when my hair grew out to the wig's length. This was my reason for wanting the shortest possible wig. Using this approach, only one obvious visible transformation would have to occur: cutting off my real hair.

THE SHEARING

A few days passed between the time I purchased my wig and scheduled an appointment to cut my hair. The salon was gracious to let me come before the store's opening hours. (Or maybe they didn't want a crybaby in the house with other customers.) Whatever the case, Susan met me once again to provide support as only a female can in such situations. I presented my wig and the stylist commenced to cutting. As he cut, I wondered if I should have waited a few weeks and shaved my head like so many cancer patients do. Parker had offered to shave his head, too, but that wasn't necessary for me. Still, I was deeply touched.

I anticipated being in tears within a few snips as I watched my long hair fall to the floor, so I was shocked to hear myself laughing and see myself smiling. There was only one explanation: the joy of the Lord giving me the strength and comfort I needed. "For the Lord God helps me, therefore, I am not disgraced" (Isa. 50:7). When it was over, I headed to work apprehensive and excited about my hair debut.

In retrospect, there were certain things I did not want to see as my hair began to detach: a bathtub drain full of hair, hair on my pillow each morning, or massive amounts of hair in my hairbrush. So I chose to cut my hair at the first sign of loosening and then thin it out myself. Often as I was driving, I would run my fingers through my hair and release a handful out of the car window. I always wondered what the driver behind me must be thinking. I got a kick out of doing that! When my hair got to the point it was time to put on the wig, my friend Sharon combed out the rest as much as possible as I sat outside in the open air. She dropped the hair onto the ground and, because it was evening, I could not see how much there was when we walked away. This unplanned strategy helped to minimize the trauma. The next day I asked Susan to trim the remaining strands in the back. From that day forward, I donned my new wig with resolve. "Blessed is a man who perseveres under trial; for once he has been approved, he will receive the crown of life, which the Lord has promised to those who love Him" (James 1:12).

Lots of cancer patients wear hats and stylish turbans; some go bald. But my wig became part of my daily wardrobe for the next eight months. I rarely took it off except when I was alone or at bedtime. I considered a cheap night wig so Parker wouldn't wake up to a scary creature, but I realized a sleeping cap (one with the fewest seams in it) was a comfortable compromise. Hats were nice for special occasions, quick trips, and yard work. I was most appreciative of my sister Elaine who eagerly provided a vast assortment of fashionable hats in different shapes, styles, and colors.

MY SACRIFICE OF PRAISE

Losing my hair seemed so senseless to me. It was very difficult to accept its loss. One night around 2 A.M., I was awakened by God's prompting. I arose and went into another room to pray. I cried and prayed until I physically hurt, attempting to reach a level of acceptance. In the midst of my prayers, the root of my problem dawned on me: there was no purpose. It was senseless to lose my hair but only if there was no purpose. I needed a purpose, a reason, something more than just a side effect. And who better to provide one than God? I stopped crying, stunned at the depth of my uncovered truth. I would turn my hair loss into a sacrifice of praise—a sacrifice to glorify God and give meaning to something I could not otherwise accept. "I urge you therefore, brethren, by the mercies of God to present your bodies a living and holy sacrifice, acceptable to God, which is your spiritual service of worship" (Rom. 12:1). I asked God to allow me to glorify him not only then, but in the future through my singing, as I desired to sing with greater confidence and conviction. From that point forward, my hair loss became meaningful and tolerable. My singing has since evolved to include an element of reverent vitality. The natural joy exudes from my being when I sing, giving praise to my God. People tell me they enjoy watching me sing as much as they enjoy listening to me sing. Whenever I hear comments like that, I remember my sacrifice of praise and think to myself, *It's God. It's all God.* "Through Him then, let us continually offer up a sacrifice of praise to God, that is, the fruit of lips that give thanks to His name. And do not neglect doing good and sharing; for with such sacrifices God is pleased" (Heb. 13:15–16).

> It was senseless to lose my hair but only if there was no purpose.

Soon after my hair began to grow back, a friend from church, Jan Storey, volunteered to give me a makeover. Jan's extra-short punk-style hair was not much longer than mine. Reluctantly, I gave in to her pleas to take off my wig and let her "do her thing." Out came gadgets, hair products, and makeup creams I didn't know existed; but by the time Jan finished "stylin' me up," I felt like a million dollars. I walked into choir rehearsal that night amid clapping and cheers. Whatever uneasiness I felt before was now transformed into prideful glamour. Jan's hair tips and putty gave me a sense of welcome newness. "Be renewed in the spirit of your mind, and put on the new self, which in the likeness of God has been created in righteousness and holiness of the truth" (Eph. 4:24–25).

Meditative Thought

What sacrifice of praise can you offer God today?

This lesson is dedicated with overflowing love to my mother, Margaret Evans O'Kelley, who will, to me, forever be the epitome of timeless beauty in spirit, heart, and body. I thank God for giving her the grace and courage to stand strong during my cancer trials.

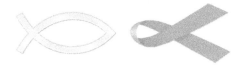

THE SHOCKS DON'T STOP

Many are the afflictions of the righteous; but the Lord delivers him out of them all.
—Psalm 34:19

Earthquakes are one of the most frightening and destructive phenomena of nature. The earthquake is traumatic enough but what follows is significant. Landslides, collapsed buildings and highways, volcanic eruptions, fires, and tsunamis are all potential after-effects from an earthquake. Aftershocks, though not as severe as the earthquake itself, can continue for months, adding to the destruction.

Though a bit melodramatic, cancer can be compared to an earthquake in that there are aftershocks all along the way. You might logically think that once a cancer diagnosis has been delivered, the shock would eventually be absorbed and subside. But that's not true. The diagnosis, or "earthquake," if you will, is just the beginning. The aftershocks are yet to come.

GET SET FOR SETBACKS

Every cancer patient has their own unique list of shocks and setbacks. They occur throughout the journey, offering new challenges. This lesson describes some of my shocks and setbacks and comes with a warning. If you prefer, you may skip today's lesson and pick up with tomorrow's.

You've already read about my most devastating shock: hair loss. The chemo-induced menopause was also an unpleasant surprise. But there were numerous other shocks and setbacks. Some of them were physical, some emotional, some medical, some even perceived—but all of them were real to me at the time.

One unanticipated shock followed surgery. My underarm was numb—for months. Nobody ever told me to expect that. Nor did they tell me I would have a drainage tube inserted in my armpit for a few days. Ever try to take a shower and wash your hair with one hand while holding a drainage bag in the other? Bandages—I didn't anticipate bandages being such an ordeal, but they stuck to my skin like a postage stamp on a letter and had to be peeled away in teeny, tiny pieces. What a shock to see what was underneath: stitches, bruising, disfigurement, and enough iodine to stain a small table.

About a week after surgery, I developed a seroma, a fluid-filled pocket. I woke up one morning with a huge soft pocket under my arm. For about two weeks, it felt conspicuous as if I were carrying the

Sunday morning newspaper under my arm. The seroma got bigger, but I never had to have it drained. It eventually reabsorbed.

Months later, I made the unsettling discovery I couldn't stretch my arm over my head. It bothered me so much that I made it my mission to remedy the situation at all painful costs. Why had I not been told to exercise my arm? I grimaced, clenching my teeth as I forced my arm to the floor a little more each day. Within a few weeks, I could lay my arm flat stretched completely over my head. It didn't feel good, still doesn't, but by golly, it was flat on the floor.

Lymphadema, what's that? I thought. It kept coming up in the mounds of reading material I had collected. *What do you mean I shouldn't shave under my arms with a razor or have my blood pressure checked and blood drawn from my surgery side for the rest of my life?* That was news to me. I felt deflated upon learning that lymphadema (swelling of the limbs) could occur at anytime throughout my entire life due to having removed numerous lymph nodes. This can be irreversible. It was almost depressing to think my arms and/or legs could blow up twice their size or bigger and stay that way. The thought became almost obsessive. After weeks, I had to finally let it go. "The Lord is good, a stronghold in the day of trouble, and He knows those who take refuge in Him" (Nah. 1:7).

There were more shocks. I was no longer considered a normal donor, which meant I could not donate blood for any purpose. Even research blood donations would have to wait until I was "normal" again. As a researcher, this cut me to the quick creating a flaw in my ongoing quest for normalcy. *Even my blood is not normal*, I thought. I did have the opportunity, however, to participate in a breast cancer intervention study. I had read about the study weeks earlier in the employee newspaper, pausing to think what a sad study it must be. Now here I was calling to enroll having met the eligibility criteria. *Perhaps my cancer could be good for something*, I sighed. The study evaluated the effects of exercise, stress management, and social support upon the immune system and well-being for breast cancer patients. I determined the regimented exercise and group support would do me good. Unfortunately, I was randomized into the control group rather than the intervention group, which meant I could not participate in the program activities. I was sorely disappointed but still agreed to participate, granting periodic blood draws and answering question-naires. I realized in retrospect, I would have never had the time to devote to the study had I been in the intervention arm. But God knew that well before I did. "My times are in Thy hand" (Ps. 31:15).

Was there a moment throughout your or your loved one's cancer journey in which you recognized God's interceding mercy?

_____

_____

DRUG REACTIONS, SORE RIBS, AND WEIGHT GAIN

One thing that never ceased to amaze me was how drugs were prescribed to counteract the side effects induced by . . . well, other drugs. This seemed ironic to me. I shuddered at the handful of prescriptions I was given to fill before my first cycle of chemotherapy. I protested the steroid but filled every one of them. One drug was low-dose coumadin (a blood thinner) for my implanted portacath. Once when I had a relentless sinus infection, I took the recommended dosage of prescribed antibiotic, only to develop a serious adverse reaction. It was later determined to have been caused from the combination of the two drugs. "Miserable" doesn't begin to describe how I felt. My back ached terribly; I had a sore throat, a mouthful of sores, sinus congestion/drainage, indigestion, and general yuckiness. Soon after taking the antibiotic, I noticed the color of my urine getting darker. It didn't take long to turn a bright red. In lab terms, I had a "4+ blood." (That's as high as it goes.) Somehow I managed to make it through the long July Fourth weekend, but I immediately brought it to the attention of the radiation staff the next workday. My coagulation level was tested and found to be critical. Dr. Nabell called in haste to have me come to the clinic for a vitamin K boost to correct the deficit. Within an hour, I felt better.

While this incident unnerved me, I was much more disturbed when I thought my cancer might have metastasized into my bones. The two occasions turned out to be false alarms. The first time was due to a slow recovery following surgery. As my body attempted to heal, the soreness moved from my neck, down to my chest, and settled in my ribs. My body, now compromised by chemotherapy, had never taken so long to heal. I could not even take a deep breath. The second scare occurred over a year later when my ribs became unusually sore again. I chalked it off to the fact I had been moving furniture, but it didn't seem right that my ribs were still sore a month later. *This is not normal. What else could it be?* I silently panicked. Fortunately, the x-rays revealed nothing abnormal and my rib pain subsided over time.

Throughout chemotherapy, I had been reading a book about a woman's journey through breast cancer. She spoke of her experiences in more detail than I was ready to absorb, so I wisely set it aside. Still, I would read a chapter here and there in conjunction with where I was in my own journey. One night I read about the effect of weight gain from the commonly prescribed post-cancer drug tamoxifen. It hit me square between my eyelash-less eyes. The author was determined not to gain weight, so she reacted by running. I reacted by crying. I had worked hard to lose weight before my diagnosis and now I would be gaining it all back? Oh, no!

One thing I learned early on was that too much information can be harmful. I stopped educating myself through the Internet, deciding I would learn first-hand as things occurred. This approach worked well. Please don't misunderstand—educating oneself is wise, but you cross a line when it causes you to become paranoid. For example, following my first cycle of chemo, I determined I had developed "chemo-brain." This is a drug-induced condition I had read about impairing one's cognitive abilities. *I surely must have it*, I thought. My speech was forced, my thoughts were spacey, my vision fuzzy, and I was "crawling out of my skin." I could barely hold a simple conversation. After mentioning the problem to my boss, I was relieved to learn it was nothing more than a reaction to the combination of anti-nausea drugs I had taken the day before. It had nothing to do with impairment of my cognitive abilities. Needless to say, Dr. Nabell changed the anti-nausea medication the next cycle, which helped.

Have you experienced any shocks or setbacks in your journey thus far? If so, briefly describe.

_____

_____

THROUGH IT ALL, THERE IS HOPE

I have divulged all of these things to demonstrate a point: there is a continuous bombardment of mind-boggling adjustments patients and loved ones must make throughout the cancer process. In truth, there were a few "good" shocks, such as the number of get-well cards I received and the number of prayer lists on which I was placed. I learned some valuable lessons through the non-stop shocks and setbacks. I learned I needed to maintain a healthy and positive mental attitude every single day. I needed God to help me do that. I learned a deeper perseverance through every shock that strengthened my relationship with God. I learned the truth of Paul's words to the people in the church in Rome. "We also exult in our tribulations, knowing that tribulation brings about perseverance; and perseverance, proven character and proven character, hope; and hope does not disappoint, because the love of God has been poured out within our hearts through the Holy Spirit who was given to us" (Rom. 5:3–5). I bet Paul never expected the vast array of aftershocks following his Christian conversion either—imprisonment; being shipwrecked, beaten, and stoned; hunger; thirst; exposure; and endangerment of life at every turn. He experienced so many shocks in his everyday Christian walk, he said, "I have learned to be content in whatever circumstances I am" (Phil. 4:11). His secret? Every day he looked to Jesus Christ, every day he persevered, and every day he bore witness to the glory of God. He never lost hope. "I can do all things through Him who strengthens me" (Phil. 4:13). You can, too.

How do you tend to respond to the shocks life brings? How should you respond?

_____

_____

_____

Life itself brings tribulations—a job loss, death of a loved one, divorce, a car accident, disappointments with children. Yet we persevere. Life moves forward. Do we still recognize God's love and His promises in the midst of those circumstances? Do we truly exult in our tribulations, like Paul, that build our character? Do we place our lives in the hope of a God who does not disappoint? Shocks and personal setbacks are here to stay, but there is an answer. "Consider it all joy, my brethren, when you encounter various trials, knowing that the testing of your faith produces endurance. And let endurance have its perfect result, that you may be perfect and complete, lacking in nothing" (James 1:2–4).

Meditative Thought

What are some shocks/setbacks in your life that have challenged you to develop perseverance and character? Do you or did you have hope through it all?

This lesson is dedicated to my dear friend and former choir buddy, Jimmie Baker. As a fellow medical technologist and breast cancer survivor, I appreciated her candid honesty and willingness to let me discuss shocking issues.

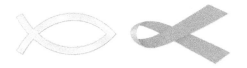

RELATIONSHIPS MOLDED

There is a friend who sticks closer than a brother.

—Proverbs 18:24

Some contend we are who we are by what we eat. Some say we are who we are by how we spend our money. Still others believe we are who we are by the lifestyle we choose. Let's consider for this lesson we are who we are by the company we keep. No doubt relationships characterize us and give us a form of unique identity. I am my husband's wife, my mother's daughter, my boss's employee, my friend's adviser, my nieces' aunt, and my dogs' caretaker. Some relationships are serious, some casual; some are dictated, some chosen. But the usual relationships don't stop there for the cancer patient. New and unfamiliar relationships emerge: patient to doctor, patient to nurse, patient to receptionist, and patient to another patient. People you've known but never realized were cancer survivors can blossom into renewed friendships. Relationships that have been stagnant for years can also become rekindled.

YOU ARE NOT ALONE

You may have already discovered that your or your loved one's cancer is not confined to just you or your loved one. Cancer concerns everyone. Sure the person with cancer has to go through the bodily effects—but it is that loved one who will be by their side. They will help bear the burden by doing distasteful things such as holding your "puke pan" or removing/changing bandages, or assist in emptying your drainage bag. Christ tells us to "bear one another's burdens, and thus fulfill the law of Christ" (Gal. 6:2). We can do that.

God created relationships so we did not have to be alone on this earth. God Himself chose not to be alone after His wondrous creation of the universe so he created man. He also created every beast of the field and every bird of the sky to cohabit with man. God looked at it and said, "It is not good for the man to be alone; I will make him a helper suitable for him" (Gen. 2:18). Thus, woman was made. So, you see, right from the start God endorsed relationships with other living creatures and beings so we might draw help and companionship from one another.

What a poignant example of love and support we see in the relationship between Ruth and her mother-in-law, Naomi. "For where you go, I will go, and where you lodge, I will lodge. Your people shall be my people, and your God, my God. Where you die, I will die, and there I will be buried. Thus may the Lord do to me, and worse, if anything but death parts you and me" (Ruth 1:16–17).

What has been one of the most treasured relationships you have had during the course of your or your loved one's cancer? Have any new relationships developed?

_____

_____

As a parent you agonize over a child's illness, wishing it somehow could be transferred to you. How I cringed to hear my loved ones say they wished they could take my place and fight my battle instead. No, never—how heart-wrenching and incredibly humbling. How could they possibly wish my cancer upon themselves? Simple: they loved me that much. "Greater love has no one than this that one lay down his life for his friends" (John 15:13).

Describe a time when you would have suffered in the place of a loved one if you could have.

_____

_____

My Greatest Concern

I was never more acutely aware of my relationships than when I was first diagnosed. Apart from my relationship with Christ, my closest relationships and how my cancer affected them mattered more to me than anything else. How would my husband deal with it? Would my widowed mother recover from her grief if I were to die? What would my nieces think? How would my sisters feel, knowing cancer was in the family now? All of these thoughts raced through my mind. My most earnest prayers were for the welfare of my loved ones. If someone asked me how they could pray for me, my response was they could pray for my loved ones. Of course I was apprehensive about what was going to happen to me, but I knew I could accept my outcome, whatever it was. What I didn't know was how my death, if it were to occur, might impact the lives of those I loved most. I didn't dwell on the issue of death, but if I could at least capture a peace about it from my loved ones, then I knew I could better accept departure from this world. I desperately wanted to know if my loved ones would be OK regardless of the outcome. It was impossible to know, yet this was how I prayed. "Hear the voice of my supplications when I cry to Thee for help, when I lift up my hands toward Thy holy sanctuary" (Ps. 28:2).

What is or was your or your loved one's greatest concern after being diagnosed with cancer?

_____

_____

LESSONS FROM A CANCER PATIENT

I came to realize that the peace I desired concerning my loved ones was dependent in part upon me. We portray ourselves through our relationships. What I mean is that others determine how we are through our interactions with them involving our attitudes, our perceived outlooks, our acceptance, and our handling of a situation. They evaluate what they can see and hear. A smile on my face must mean I am feeling OK, food on my plate indicates I can eat, and energy in my walk demonstrates I am not depressed. From what could be seen and heard, it appeared to the outside world I was coping admirably. However, the minute a discontented look appeared on my face or I was absent from church—that meant something was wrong. Therefore, it was crucial to present myself in a manner that was consoling and accepting to others. Funny thing is—it, in turn, brought consolation to me.

Another less obvious effect of the importance of our relationships is that we become a "walking lesson book." People watch how you respond to crisis. They want to know your "secret" so that if they ever have a devastating illness such as cancer they can practice what does and does not work based upon your example. What works will be tucked away in the recesses of their mind. I confess to doing that, evaluating how courageous this person was or how sad that one seemed based on the interactions I witnessed.

What is a trait or two you recall from someone you admired going through a difficult time?

THE MOST IMPORTANT RELATIONSHIP: GOD

We have already established that God gave us relationships so we don't have to go through life alone. But it's not our earthly relationships that bring salvation and supernatural comfort, peace, and joy—it's the relationship with God that does that. It is only through God where we can unload our suffering, intense desires, and innermost fears.

As Christians, it is important to mold our relationships through the one relationship that has eternal significance. If your relationship with God is on shaky ground, then your earthly relationships are probably suffering, too. But if your relationship with God is in good standing, then it will be obvious through your relationships with others. An automatic outflow of God's love and power will be evident. What a way for non-Christians to see what God can do through the devastation of cancer.

RELATIONSHIPS MOLDED

Reflecting upon the idea that cancer affects relationships, I wondered specifically how it had affected mine. I deciding to pose a question to family members and close friends: how has my cancer affected our relationship? I determined it had affected some more than others. With Parker, our relationship didn't change as much as the appreciation of it, our marriage, and of life in general. "Nothing in this world should be taken for granted," he said. My mother and I developed a richer, more open spiritual relationship, while my mother-in-law became more receptive to my suggestions concerning how to handle some of her own health issues. As for my sisters, they seemed to respect sentimentalities that otherwise would have been overlooked. My friend Susan, who suffers from chronic pain, noted that I handled pain differently from her, prompting her to delve deeper into God's Word. My friend Sharon, who witnessed her mother's year-long deterioration and subsequent death from cancer, said she had great admiration for me but had reservations that as my faith increased, death might be closer. Sharon better understands now through her own struggles that we always ought to strive for a more intimate relationship with God, regardless of the outcome.

Relationships with distant relatives and friends were rejuvenated, some graduating beyond casual contact to a more personal level. Church relationships were enhanced, particularly those with my pastor and his family as they prayed daily for me throughout my cancer ordeal. All of these relationships were impacted, but the one that was impacted the most was the one I have with Jesus Christ. My relationship with Him is eternal.

Meditative Thought

Whether you are a believer or a non-believer, how has your relationship with Jesus Christ been affected by your or your loved one's cancer?

This lesson is dedicated to my two sisters, Elaine O'Kelley Mizzell and Nancy O'Kelley Nunnelley, who reached out to me in their own loving and special ways. Their quiet and prayerful support was felt and appreciated. How I love them, their husbands, George and Henry, and my three beautiful nieces, Stephanie, Kristina, and Jennifer.

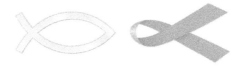

THE SHADOW OF DEATH

But encourage one another day after day, as long as it is still called "Today."
—Hebrews 3:13

Cancer. Death. Two words evoking a plethora of emotions; two words that capture the essence of fear. Are they synonymous? Do they both mean an end to life? Do we feel a silent doom when we hear of someone being diagnosed with cancer—or worse, when that someone is us? These questions are difficult to answer. There are times when we must accept that only God knows the answers.

What a delicate picture of trust we see in Martha after her brother, Lazarus, died despite her and her sister's pleas for Jesus to come. Jesus waited four days after Lazarus' death before coming. Not understanding what Jesus was about to do, Martha reaffirmed her belief in His words that "he who believes in Me shall live even if he dies."

Read John 11:20–27.
What did Jesus mean when He said, "Everyone who lives and believes in Me shall never die?"

_____

_____

As the story of Lazarus unfolds from his death to his resurrection, we see a wide array of emotions ranging from distress and grief to joy and worship—all demonstrating an underlying trust in Jesus. Let's address the same trust we can have for the same Jesus as Mary and Martha. There are two truths that ring out to me while walking in the shadow of death. First, each of us has today as indicated by our focal verse. And second, our future as believers is one of eternal bliss. We can rely upon these two truths at all times. The remainder of the lesson will focus on each truth in greater depth.

HAVING TODAY

One night as I was watching television, I became enthralled with a human interest story titled "Radical Trust" about a gentleman with end-stage cancer from my home state of Alabama. His name was James Collier. He shared some simple, yet profound observations he had made during his cancer journey. One was that his prognosis was exactly the same as anyone else's. "We all die," he said. "Each of us faces the same realities. Namely, that we have today—the joy of the present moment."[3] He's right. We do have today. Mr. Collier understands very well that "this is the day which the Lord hath made; let us rejoice and be glad in it" (Ps. 118:24).

The word *today* is no doubt a significant word to a dying person. But shouldn't *today* be an important word to all of us? Tomorrow may not bring another today. So let us do as Christ tells us to do—live today and be glad in it, savoring the joy of each precious moment. "Who of you by worrying can add a single hour to his life?" (Matt. 6:27 NIV).

What is something you can do to celebrate having today?

_____

CANCER IS NOT A DEATH SENTENCE

"Cancer is a word, not a sentence," said a cancer survivor. *How true*, I thought. I remembered the letter written by my surgeon's husband given to me on the day of my diagnosis. "You have not received a death sentence," it read. The letter further explained that millions of people in the world were far closer to death than I and that thousands had cancer and didn't even know it. Furthermore, my biopsy report did not make any difference! *What?* I thought. I read further. The letter said I was just like anybody else and would pass out of this world when the time was fulfilled. *When the time was fulfilled*, I pondered. *Would that be soon?* The letter acknowledged that although my biopsy was positive, it did not mean God was asking me to accept death now. Therefore, I should choose life with all the strength of my will and passion of my soul. *Yes, I will do that.*

> "Cancer is a word, not a sentence."

Those words encouraged me as did the Death Angel's words in the television series *Touched by an Angel*. "You will face death in the same manner you face life," the angel said.[4] *OK, then*, I rationalized. *I will face life and death with strength and courage.*

VALLEYS AND SHADOWS

"Even though I walk through the valley of the shadow of death, I fear no evil; for Thou art with me; Thy rod and Thy staff, they comfort me" (Ps. 23:4). There are at least three inferences from this verse to consider. First, there can be no valley if there is no mountain. I envision Christ coming down from the mountaintop into the valley to walk with us.

Second, notice the verse says "through" the valley as if we are heading somewhere. We won't always be in the valley; but for now, the valley is a passage of twists, turns, and streams to be forged. The valley is a vulnerable place, a place of fear—a legitimate fear that warrants protection. But we need not allow fear to overshadow the confidence we can have in our Protector. "In the fear of the Lord there is strong confidence, and his children will have refuge" (Prov. 14:26).

The third inference is there can be no shadow if there is no light. A shadow can only be cast in the presence of light. Christ is our light. The shadow is created not only by the light but also by the object that is in the light. A shadow cannot overtake the object; but it can change in size, depending on where the object is placed in the light and the angle that the light is shining upon it. In Psalm 23, death has not yet come to the psalmist. However, the shadow follows him wherever he goes. And wherever the shadow goes, reasoning tells us there is light. "For Thou dost light my lamp; the Lord my God illumines my darkness" (Ps. 18:28).

Why do you think the psalmist was comforted by "Thy rod and Thy staff"?

_____

_____

FOCUSING ON HIS KINGDOM

Ken Hemphill, author of *The Prayer of Jesus*, says, "When we attempt to manage our own kingdom affairs, we become anxious because we have no power to control our circumstances. Jesus understands this limitation and presents to us an offer we should be unable to refuse: you focus on my Kingdom and I, in turn, will manage yours."[5]

A few months following the completion of my cancer treatments, Parker and I were awakened one night to the flashing lights of emergency vehicles outside our window. We knew it was not a good sign as our neighbor had been battling cancer for eight years and had not been doing well. We learned the next day that Susan Cook had died peacefully during the night. She was close to my age. We had shared "cancer stories" a few weeks earlier. We laughed as she told me how my dog Skippy would come visit her in her bedroom and curl up beside her on the bed. Now here I was about to attend her funeral. I was not prepared.

At the close of the service, I made my way to the front to speak to Susan's husband. I saw Susan's oncologist and nurse, who happened to also be my oncologist and nurse, waiting to speak to the family, too. None of us could hold back the tears as each of us shared and reflected upon our own unique relationship with Susan and to one another. "Precious in the sight of the Lord is the death of His godly ones" (Ps. 116:15).

Through eight long years and three cancer recurrences, Susan delayed death and exemplified what it meant to "have today." She ushered in each new day with an eternal perspective. She kissed her husband each morning as he went to work and hugged her son as he met the school bus, knowing it might be her last day on this earth. I wondered how she could do that. "I will praise the Lord while I live; I will sing praises to my God while I have my being" (Ps. 146:2).

The description the pastor gave at the funeral of how Susan lived was this: not with regrets but with hope, not with sorrow but with resurrection, and not with bitterness but with love. Susan had learned to embrace both life and death with strength and passion, knowing that a life in Christ is worthwhile and that our home is not here on earth. "For our citizenship is in heaven, from which also we eagerly wait for a Savior, the Lord Jesus Christ" (Phil 3:20).

What is something that you can do today that will have eternal significance?

_____

_____

A Future of Eternal Bliss

"We live in the land of the dying and are heading to the land of the living," said an unknown source. For a Christian, death is an entrance into eternal bliss with God. We die in His sight and in His time—not alone, randomly or accidentally, but embraced by His arms of mercy and love. When you stop to think about it, death is for our benefit. The Bible says, "The day of one's death is better than the day of one's birth" (Eccl. 7:1). We shall be free from pain in death, we shall gain perfect wisdom, we shall experience eternal reunion with our loved ones, and; best of all, we shall enjoy the presence of God, having been made in His likeness. Eternal bliss? I'd say so.

Meditative Thought

After reading this lesson, have you changed your viewpoint of cancer and death? If so, how?

This lesson is dedicated to the memory of Susan Cook, who fought a long, hard battle with cancer, living every day in the joy of the present.

Week 5

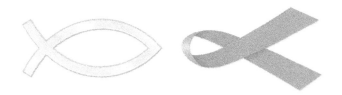

THE PROCESS:
THE RESPONSES

As we enter the last week of "The Process," I hope you have found some helpful nuggets along the way to build your faith through the trials of cancer. I am excited about this upcoming week's lessons as we move into "The Responses." You will be challenged to make decisions as to how you will respond to the diagnosis, plan, and effects cancer has had upon you. You may also come to recognize your role in God's plan for your life through this experience. It is my hope during this week of faith-building lessons that you will find a freedom from the burdens cancer brings. Join me in exploring outlets of release, ways to build faith, worshiping God regardless of circumstances, finding peace, and stepping into the "glory zone."

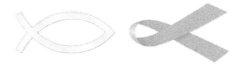

FINDING AN OUTLET

The Lord is my rock and my fortress and my deliverer, my God, my rock, in whom I take refuge.
—Psalm 18:2

How exciting to reach the heart of our study, where we will examine positive responses to cancer you can choose to make. Making choices can be a rare privilege to a cancer patient who must yield to an ongoing loss of control including not being able to use your time as you did before since much of it is spent in treatment or recovering from it; not eating the same foods you used to eat because many of them now make you nauseated, are too difficult to chew, or are too hard to swallow; not having the energy to perform routine activities; not being able to do things by yourself; and one of the most helpless, feeling as if your body is no longer your own. How you respond to this and more is something you as a cancer patient or one who has been touched by the effects of cancer have control over. They are not easy choices but, nonetheless, they are undeniably a choice.

You have come to a crossroads—a place where your decisions can affect the rest of your life, a place for evaluating your strength and belief systems. The truth with which you have now come face to face with is how you will respond to God. What you decide reveals what you believe about Him. Read that last sentence again and write that statement below, inserting the word *I* instead of *you*.

_____

Do you trust what God says in His Word enough to put it into practice? Do you believe He is in control when everything appears to be in disarray? You decide. "'And if it is disagreeable in your sight to serve the Lord, choose for yourselves today whom you will serve; whether the gods which your fathers served which were beyond the River, or the gods of the Amorites in whose land you are living; but as for me and my house, we will serve the Lord'" (Josh. 24:15).

OUTLETS OF CHOICE

Choosing God to be your primary outlet to the cancer affecting your life is your best recourse. Besides, you will end up finding an outlet of some sort sooner or later. Reading, camping, and working puzzles are examples of outlets, but I found satisfaction and worth in any outlet that recognized God and His attributes. I discovered that when I incorporated God into my outlet, the result was more profitable. Below are some of my outlets and their results. Use them to develop some of your own outlets.

MUSIC: AN OUTLET OF EMOTIONS

The Result: Greater Intimacy with God

I love music, both instrumental and vocal. Music has always been a significant part of my life. It has a way of tapping into my emotions to provide release or to create a bridge to be more open with God. Some of my most memorable encounters with God involve music. There were times during my journey of faith when I was too weak or too distraught to pray that music itself became my prayer. In contrast, I have been so full of joy at times that music has been used to express my exhilaration. A few times I have felt as if my heart were singing. Music often becomes a voice for my emotions.

David was an example of how music can serve as an outlet. The book of Psalms, which was a hymnal for the Jews, refers many times to David's music in celebration to God. "My heart is steadfast, O God; I will sing, I will sing praises, even with my soul" (Ps. 108:1). David also made instruments solely for this purpose. "And the priests stood at their posts and the Levites, with the instruments of music to the Lord, which King David had made for giving praise to the Lord" (2 Chron. 7:6). David's skillful harp playing gave him an opportunity to play for King Saul upon his summons. Read 1 Samuel 16:14–23 to see why David's music was important to King Saul.

What did David's music do for King Saul?

_____

List some specific songs that have a positive emotional impact on you.

_____

_____

Did you know there is now scientific proof validating music as an outlet to stress? It's true. Music helps boost the immune system and serves as a muscle relaxant. Certain parts of the brain are triggered, creating a lingering positive impact emotionally and physically. In his book, *Messenger of Paradise*, Charles Levinthal explains how listening to music releases endorphins that relieve pain and induce euphoria. A study conducted at Temple University discovered that listening to music for twenty minutes significantly elevated one's IgA, a disease-fighting antibody normally found in the body.[1] So turn on the music!

SINGING AND PLAYING INSTRUMENTS: AN OUTLET OF PRAISE

The Result: Joy

Throughout my journey of faith, as I was able, I welcomed the opportunity to sing or play the piano or organ because God had put a new song in my heart and I wanted to share it. "Sing to Him a new song; play skillfully with a shout of joy" (Ps. 33:3). While it is not unusual for me to sing or play instruments, I felt my circumstances at the time lent themselves to greater witness and, therefore, greater glory to God. Since having cancer, I have learned to better express my joy to God, singing to Him rather than to an audience.

CARING PEOPLE: AN OUTLET OF NEED

The Result: Reassurance

Support is crucial during times of crisis. It is never more important than when you reach your melting point. Mine came soon after starting chemotherapy. Parker called me at work one day to tell me he needed to readmit his mother to the hospital. It sounded serious. However, I had troubles of my own. I knew when I got home I would have a hard time walking the dogs without his help. I was still recovering from surgery and unable to fully use my left arm.

It was also around this time I needed to make a decision about my hair. It would be falling out soon. I wanted to go ahead and get it cut, but I needed to decide on a hairstyle. I stopped by the grocery store on my way home and bought two hairstyle magazines. As I got back in the car, I felt a panic attack coming on. I had never experienced a panic attack before but had witnessed a few. All at once, I didn't want to be alone. Parker was gone and wouldn't be home until later that night. I couldn't face the severity of my mother-in-law's health issues in addition to my own. What if she were dying? How could I support my husband during my own time of need? Plus, I was about to be bald. The panic was taking hold. I was melting fast like butter in a hot pan.

I called my friend, Dr. Paula Moore, who lived nearby. I knew she would understand both as a friend and a doctor. When Paula answered the phone, I could barely speak as I choked back the tears. She sensed my immediate need and agreed to meet me at home. She was waiting on the deck with my dogs when I pulled in the driveway. We walked the dogs together and spent the next few hours in conversation and prayer as God used her in a mighty way to speak peace into every concern I had. Paula's confidence, knowledge, and reassurance were God's prescription for me that day. As a mother of three, including a special needs child whom she was in the process of bathing when I called, Paula and her husband, Darrell, made a sacrifice for me that will not soon be forgotten. "A friend loves at all times, and a brother is born for adversity" (Prov. 17:17).

Have you experienced a meltdown during this cancer journey or any other time? How did you handle it?

_____

_____

_____

WORSHIP: AN OUTLET OF GRATITUDE AND SUBMISSION

The result: Humility

Having learned that God enters into my pain and shares it with me, worship became a time of gratitude. Only God could love me with such a love that He would willingly enter into my pain. Even in my physical and emotional frailty, I recognized the need to offer reverent thanks. "In everything give thanks; for this is God's will for you in Christ Jesus" (1 Thess. 5:18).

Worship also reinforced my attitude of submission. I often needed to be reminded I was not alone and my cancer was not my own. Worship did that for me. It helped me retain the focus of seeking God on a more intimate level. Submitting to God every day was both necessary and relieving. I knew in my heart God would walk with me every step of the way, but I needed a constant reminder. A cycle of submission and gratitude birthed greater humility that responded with submission and gratitude. "The reward of humility and the fear of the Lord are riches, honor and life" (Prov. 22:4).

BIBLE READING: AN OUTLET OF SEEKING

The Result: Encouragement and Comfort

"O Lord, Thou hast searched me and known me. Thou dost know when I sit down and when I rise up; Thou dost understand my thought from afar. Thou dost scrutinize my path and my lying down, and art intimately acquainted with all my ways" (Ps. 139:1–3). I needed to read those words after my biopsy and then again after my diagnosis. I needed to know God knew me better than I did because that meant He also knew my cancer and the effect it had on my loved ones. I wanted Him to scrutinize my path and be deeply acquainted with my ways because He had already blazed the trail.

I love how familiar verses take on a fresh meaning in different circumstances of life. It's one of the ways God speaks to us. Psalm 23:4 became more real to me than ever. "Even though I walk through the valley of the shadow of death, I fear no evil; for Thou art with me; Thy rod and Thy staff, they comfort me." As the verse says, I felt as though I was walking through the valley of the shadow of death, yet I was able to find comfort, encouragement, and companionship. How could this be? Because with Christ there is no evil in death or even its shadow, only comfort.

PRAISE: AN OUTLET OF ESCAPE

The Result: Freedom

There were times I wanted my adrenalin-pumping brain to take a break and stop thinking about cancer. "Will I ever stop thinking about it?" I asked a seven-year cancer survivor. "Yes," she said emphatically. But for the present time, praising God was the only sure way to relieve my obsession as I placed my focus and energy solely upon God and away from myself for that designated moment. Needless to say, I did this often. It was difficult at first but became easier. It was so freeing. What's more, it was sweet and glorifying to God. "Now the Lord is the Spirit; and where the Spirit of the Lord is, there is liberty" (2 Cor. 3:17).

PRAYER: AN OUTLET OF DESPERATION

The Result: Peace

Prayer was, and still is, the best outlet of them all. I could pour out my heart day or night and God, in His state of constant attentiveness, would always hear. "He who keeps Israel will neither slumber nor sleep" (Ps. 121:4). Oftentimes during the night I awakened to seek reassurance from God, which He gladly gave. "I will bless the Lord who has counseled me; indeed, my mind instructs me in the night" (Ps. 16:7).

Prayer is a spiritual flow. Talking to God is more than just talking to a person. You are conversing with the great I Am, someone who is genuinely interested in what you have to say. Even if you are angry it's OK to release your emotions and desperation into His capable hands. The creator of the universe can handle your anger and frustration. "Be anxious for nothing, but in everything by prayer and supplication with thanksgiving let your requests be made known to God" (Phil. 4:6). Not only is prayer a means of release but prayer changes us, not God, to make our hearts and minds more like His.

Prayers from friends who not only prayed *for* me but *with* me gave me great comfort and delight. My friend Theresa Nolen offered to come to my house before my surgery to have a time of praise, worship, and prayer. It was a stretch out of her comfort zone and mine but was a tremendous blessing providing a much-needed outlet. Theresa's prayers lingered in my mind as I sat in the radiology room a few days later being prepped for surgery. Once again, her prayers brought me great comfort.

How has cancer affected your prayer life?

_____

_____

Pat Sullivan, Heisman trophy winner and 1994 Southwest Conference Coach of the Year, said of prayer after his cancer diagnosis: "You can get down on your knees and pray or you can give up. I didn't pray to be healed; I just prayed to be given some peace, to be able to handle whatever I was facing."[2] I completely understand. A handwritten statement in my Bible from an unknown source says, "Peace comes in the proportion to your needs and to your will to have it." I believe that is true. "The steadfast of mind Thou wilt keep in perfect peace, because he trusts in Thee" (Isa. 26:3). Oh, Lord, may we trust You to bring us that perfect peace.

Summarization of My Outlets

Mode	Expression	Result
music	emotions	greater intimacy with God
singing/playing	praise	joy
caring people	need	reassurance
worship	gratitude, submission	humility
Bible reading	seeking	encouragement, comfort
praise	escape	freedom
prayer	desperation	peace

Meditative Thought

Identify at least three outlets you can use in dealing with your or your loved one's cancer.

This lesson is dedicated to the memory of Aline Evans, who succumbed to breast cancer years ago. Though she is absent from the body, her legacy lives on as a devoted church pianist in my hometown church of First Baptist Church in Sylacauga, Alabama.

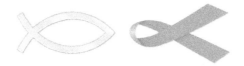

BUILDING THE FAITH

If we are faithless, He remains faithful; for He cannot deny Himself.
—2 Timothy 2:13

You know the old cliché: Be careful what you pray for because you just might get it! I bet we all have testimonies to validate the truth of that statement. One thing we fail to recognize, however, is that we only get what we ask for when it falls within God's will. A few months before my cancer diagnosis, I prayed to increase my faith. I wanted a deeper faith, one that reached beyond me toward others to a more noticeable degree. I asked God to teach me how to have that kind of faith. Little did I know it would soon come under the guise of cancer!

FAITH IS A RESPONSE

Beth Moore, Christian author and speaker, says, "Faith is a response; not an action. If we strive to have faith, we may be miserably disappointed. But if we learn to trust in His faithfulness, we will be greatly blessed."[3]

We cannot always choose what happens to us, but we can choose how we will respond to a situation. I chose to respond to my cancer in a way that would build my faith. Let me emphasize that I didn't wrestle with keeping my faith—I wanted to build my faith. "God expects more than just perseverance in our faith; we need to build it," my Sunday school teacher said. I felt confident in the assurance that my faith would keep me and sustain me, but I longed for more than just sustenance. A sustain pedal on a piano sustains only what has been played. However, I didn't want just the lingering effects of my faith—I wanted a "chord-building" new kind of faith, something with intensity and foundational substance.

I came to the conclusion that if I were going to be presented with the massive challenge of cancer from which to build my faith, then I wanted to pass the test with flying colors. I surely didn't want to take this test again!

Read James 1:2–4 (NASB) and fill in the blanks.
"The testing of your faith produces _____. And let _____ have its _____ result, that you may be _____ and _____, lacking in nothing."

MEASURES OF FAITH

The degree of our faithfulness is directly related to our belief in God's believability. We need not become self-absorbed in quantifying the amount of faith we have even though the disciples themselves asked Jesus to "increase our faith" (Luke 17:5). Below are some examples describing a measure of faith and the result:

	Measure	Result
2 Thessalonians 1:3	_____	_____
Acts 14:8–10	_____	_____
1 Timothy 4:1	_____	_____
Matthew 17:18–20	_____	_____
Luke 17:6	_____	_____

As you can see, faith as small as a mustard seed can go a long way but let's take it a step further. In the book *God Is in Control*, Charles Stanley says God isn't satisfied with a little faith or a lot of faith; He wants perfect faith. What then, is perfect faith?

> Little Faith says, "Oh, I know He can. Will He? I know He can."
> Great Faith says, "I know He can and hallelujah, I know He will."
> Perfect Faith says, "It's as good as done. God made the promise."

We may have little faith; we may have great faith. God isn't as interested in how much faith we have as He is in that what we have is perfect. As I was writing this lesson, I received an e-mail from a friend who wanted me to know of her prayers concerning this study. She told me, "Once I have touched and agreed, it is done until the Lord comes." Now that's perfect faith.

In developing my own layman's definition of perfect faith, I came to the understanding that perfect faith is the acceptance of waiting and allowing God to be God. Perfect faith is in no way passive. It is a blend of active patience and passionate pursuit while seeking God's heart in the midst of surrender. Patience is hard work that brings about change within our hearts. The acceptance that follows is nestled in perfect faith accompanied by its intended purpose.

THE PURPOSE AND PRACTICE OF FAITH

The purpose of faith is not to change our circumstances as much as we may want it to; the purpose of faith is to change us. Remember faith is about our response—a response to God, which is a direct correlation to the relationship we have with Him, a relationship deepened by the intimacy we develop through a living fellowship.

I have learned, and am still reminded, that putting faith into practice does not always feel good. Let's compare it to a new pair of shoes that must be worn for a while before being broken in. There may be times when we have to fight to maintain our faith. Paul referred to this "good fight" in 2 Timothy 4:7. "I have fought the good fight, I have finished the course, I have kept the faith."

Why do we need to fight for our faith? One of Satan's most effective weapons is fear. It is easy to have fear in the face of cancer. Destructive fear, in contrast to wise fear (the kind your parents taught you), is a product of the power of darkness. Satan will stop at nothing to create an atmosphere where fear abounds, but we can combat that by fighting the good fight and keeping the faith.

Read Psalm 3.
What was David's solution to his fear?

_____

_____

After giving it some prayerful thought, what is your solution to any fears you may have concerning your or your loved one's cancer?

_____

_____

Be encouraged that just like the new shoes that aren't comfortable at first, the more you wear them, the more comfortable they become. Soon we find we want to wear them more and more. Similarly, the more we put our faith into practice, the more it begins to take residence within our hearts.

A Twist of Faith

Jesus said, "Have faith in God" (Mark 11:22). Sounds easy for the believer. How then, can we distort such a simple mandate? Let's examine two ways: by putting faith in faith itself and by attaching superstitious thinking to faith. You may be saying to yourself, "But I don't do that." Are you sure?

My friend Pastor B.R. Johnson, author of *Simple Living in a Complex World*, explains the concept of putting faith in faith itself:

> Faith must always have an object. Throughout the Bible the object of faith was God—His power, His work, and more. But there were those who instead of putting their faith in God placed it in a practice (Acts 14:8–10). Today we can have faith in an experience or ritual that makes us feel comfortable and maybe even spiritual, yet not be placing our faith in God. Rituals certainly have meaning but only as long as they do not replace the relationship we have with God.
>
> When I live my Christian life in a reliance on the faith working in times past and not desiring or seeking the freshness of God each and every day, then I am placing my faith in the faith that I have and not in God. The object of my faith becomes faith itself. We have lost the awesome reverence and holiness of God in our lives and tend to coast from day to day with a comfortable feeling. Just because I have faith and have expressed my faith in the past having earnestly sought God, I must not live on the past experiences but must seek Him on a daily basis.[4]

Christian author and speaker, Marilyn Meberg, explains superstitious faith:

> Maybe the reason I got an unexpected check for one hundred dollars is that I've been reading my Bible more. Or maybe the reason my health is poor is because I have not been praying enough, or tithing enough. These are not faith-based thoughts. These are superstitious thoughts. Superstitious thinking leads me to believe that if I improve my acts of "good works," then I will win more of God's favor. As a result, my circumstances will get better. On the other hand, when things go awry, there must be something I'm doing wrong. When I think like this, I am reducing God to a good-luck charm that can be rubbed when I need him.[5]

Has there ever been a time when you have experienced a twist of faith like either of these examples? Explain.

_____

_____

THE SIDE EFFECTS OF FAITH

As we learned, we need to place our focus on God—not our faith, not anointings, not a physician, not trying to determine what you or your loved one did to deserve cancer, but solely upon God. Cancer absolutely cannot be the focus, although that is what our human nature screams. Let me say that again: cancer cannot be the focus. Repeat that three times out loud. Listen to yourself say it. Allow your focus to be the vehicle that brings you to that place of perfect faith. "Set your mind on the things above, not on the things that are on earth" (Col. 3:2). Strive to have patience while you actively pursue a deeper intimacy with God as you willingly surrender to His plan for your life, whatever that plan may be.

It takes discipline—more discipline than you think—but you will be rewarded not only spiritually, but physically, and mentally. I confess there were times when I would lose my focus. Those were the times when I literally could feel the heaviness of my burdens bearing down on me. My body felt heavier, my walk became slower, my thoughts were dulled, and my energy level was drained like water evaporating from a steam iron. The plight of my circumstances caused me to falter when I would focus on them but when I would redirect my focus toward God, these symptoms would disappear. My energy revived (as much as it could), my walk became normal, my thoughts cleared, and my body lightened.

FUNDING FAITH

I found it surprising and interesting that the federal government seems to at least be recognizing and investigating the realm of faith as a major factor in health education and in the health of individuals. The National Cancer Institute has funded research at the institution where I work to determine if a spiritually based breast cancer communication project is more effective than a secular communication program among African-American female churchgoers. The overall theme of the study encourages women not only to trust in God but also to take charge of their health through preventive care and to share what they learn with others. Bible verses are used as an intervention tool along with booklets featuring several spiritual topics. Perhaps the results will unveil to non-Christians that which Christians already know: faith matters.

Meditative Thought

What can you do to move toward achieving a more perfect faith?

This lesson is dedicated to my devoted and courageous friend Sharon Atwood, whose incredible faith, forgiveness, and compassionate spirit are demonstrated in her daily living. In her own way, she prepared me to face my cancer long before it ever happened.

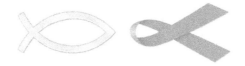

WORSHIP GOD ANYWAY

For as long as life is in me, and the breath of God is in my nostrils,
my lips certainly will not speak unjustly, nor will my tongue mutter deceit.
—Job 27:3–4

Worshiping God comes natural for believers. It's what we do in church. It's what we do in the beauty of a majestic landscape or the spectacular colors of fall. It's easy to worship God when we can visually see His handiwork. It's easy when we see His favorable intervention in our lives, such as a better job or a house that finally sells. But what about when we can't see His handiwork or we don't understand His seeming lack of compassion? What about when an unexpected death occurs or when your dream has been shattered? How about when your health has been compromised? Do you worship God then? Is there praise in your heart? The lesson today is a very important one—perhaps the most important lesson in the entire study. If you gain nothing else, harvest the gold of "worshiping God anyway."

TRAIN YOUR BRAIN

Not only is worship a recognition of God's sovereignty, it is an act of obedience. Jesus said in Luke 4:8, "You shall worship the Lord your God and serve Him only." There are no stipulations as to when we are to worship. It says to worship, straight up. Our environment, finances, health, and circumstances should not dictate if or when we worship. Look at Job's words of praise in our focal verse—and he had some major problems!

One of the positive aspects of worship is that it keeps us focused on God and not on ourselves. When we set our minds on ourselves and the things of this earth, we inevitably find disappointment and failure. However, when we set our minds on God, our perspective is kept where it needs to be: God first, everything else second. "For the mind set on the flesh is death, but the mind set on the Spirit is life and peace . . ." (Rom. 8:6).

Glorifying His name is our primary reason for existence on this earth. Therefore, we are to worship God at all times—through the good, the bad, the hard, the sad, the lovely, and the ugly. Nothing or no thing is exempt—even the trees of the field. "For you will go out with joy, and be led forth with peace; the mountains and the hills will break forth into shouts of joy before you, and all the trees of the field will clap their hands" (Isa. 55:12).

Another aspect of worship is that it is not reliant on feelings; it is an act of faith and obedience. Feelings are a manifestation of emotion, and worship does not have to coincide with emotion. In fact, worship out of feelings is shallow. It doesn't have to *feel* right—it is right!

Indicate below the times when you have been prone to worship God.

_____ during a performance of the *Messiah*

_____ during a funeral

_____ when your car that you just paid off is wrecked

_____ during stand-still traffic on the freeway

_____ listening to an inspirational sermon

_____ receiving difficult news about a loved one's health

_____ trying to meet the crunch of a deadline

You get the idea. It's not how we feel at any given moment. It's how we respond. We don't feel like worshiping God when we receive heart-stopping news that a loved one was drowned in a flash flood. We don't tend to fall to our knees in praise when the car won't start. No, we are not prone to worship God at all times, but we can strive to train our brains to let Him be our first thought of the morning and to seek His purpose and opportunities throughout the day in our ups and downs. "Rejoice always; pray without ceasing; in everything give thanks; for this is God's will for you in Christ Jesus" (1 Thess. 5:16–18).

Don't Forget to Remember

Worshiping God through the difficult moments in life requires us to remember. What do I mean? By remembering what His Word says, or recalling past experiences when we could see His hand, we can cling to these things to help us through our present difficulties. The word *remember* is used over 150 times in the Bible. *The New International Encyclopedia of Bible Words* refers to the Old Testament's call to remember as more than an invitation to think about the past. It is a call to identify oneself with the past and to let the present be shaped by it.[6]

What are some things you can remember about God when you are going through the fiery furnace?

_____

_____

Among the things I like to remember are His promises, His attributes, how much He loves and cares for me, how much He thinks about me, and how He knows my heart.

Let's examine Psalm 73. Asaph, King David's appointed minister of music, develops an envious heart as he looks on the wealthy wicked and not on God. He compares his woes to the easy increase in the wicked man's wealth. Not until Asaph comes into the sanctuary and sees the truth does he recapture his faith in God and realizes the foolishness of his ways. Asaph remembers God upon returning to the sanctuary. Could there be a lesson there for us? "It was troublesome in my sight until I came into the sanctuary of God; then I perceived their end. But as for me, the nearness of God is my good; I have made the Lord God my refuge, that I may tell of all Thy works" (Ps. 73:16–17, 28).

Habakkuk is another example of how we need to remember God. Habakkuk doesn't understand why God allows wicked practices and condemnation of the righteous to continue in the land of Judah. He questions God who responds by telling him to write His prophetic response on tablets so others may read and understand it. In the end, Habakkuk praises God, remembering who He is, His power, and His purpose. He moves from asking "why" to wonder to worship and proclaims his faith in the final verses of the book. "Though the fig tree should not blossom, and there be no fruit on the vines, though the yield of the olive should fail, and the fields produce no food, though the flock should be cut off from the fold, and there be no cattle in the stalls, yet I will exult in the Lord, I will rejoice in the God of my salvation" (Hab. 3:17–18).

A third example comes from Psalm 42 as the writer, exiled in Palestine, yearns to return to the temple in Jerusalem. "O my God, my soul is in despair within me; therefore I remember Thee from the land of the Jordan, and the peaks of Hermon, from Mount Mizar" (Ps. 42:6). His remembrance leads him back to worship.

To tie it all together, the New Testament's call to remember reinforces the Old Testament's call through the remembrance of the Lord's Supper. "Do this in remembrance of me" (1 Cor. 11:24). The Lord's Supper invites us to remember Jesus' crucifixion and identify ourselves with Him reminding us of why we are to worship.

The Lord's Supper is a symbol of Jesus' sacrificial death for our sins. Perhaps you can create a symbolic act to remind you of God's nearness (listen to a special song, hum a tune, have a dedicated place of meditation, burn a candle). List your symbolic act(s):

How Can I Worship Thee? Let Me Count the Ways

As Parker and I proudly hung our newly purchased Thomas Kinkade painting above our mantle, I removed some papers from the back to put in a secure place. A statement caught my eye. Kinkade was describing the purpose of his painting: "The impulse to worship is not confined within the vaulted ceiling and colored windows of a church." I studied the intricate details of the Dogwood Chapel painting. It seemed such a cozy place in which to worship—a stone-built chapel with colorful stained glass windows nestled in the misty mountains amid pink and white dogwoods. A gentle stream flowed under the arched bridge with lily pads and flittering butterflies. *It would be easy to worship there*, I thought. But the impulse to worship must not come from our surroundings—it must come from a faithful heart. This is especially true when our surroundings are composed of hurt, pain, sorrow, fear, and uncertainty. We need to rally alongside the psalmist, proclaiming, "I will give Thee thanks with all my heart; though I walk in the midst of trouble, Thou wilt revive me; Thou wilt stretch forth Thy hand against the wrath of my enemies, and Thy right hand will save me. The Lord will accomplish what concerns me" (Ps. 138:1, 7–8).

Worship is not confined to a church sanctuary—it can happen in an office, car, home, or at the kitchen sink. It can occur in unlikely places. Remember the radiation treatment room? I have worshiped

God in a bubbly bathtub, under a sterile bio-safety cabinet, and in a roomful of noisy people. In the movie *Facing the Giants*, worship occurred in a football locker room as the team praised God for their victories and losses. Church services, music, offerings, Bible reading, prayer, and praise are only some of the ways to evoke a spirit of worship—we should never put limits on it. Wherever the place, whenever the moment, whatever the situation, let us worship God. "Come, let us worship and bow down; let us kneel before the Lord our Maker" (Ps. 95:6).

> Wherever the place, whenever the moment, whatever the situation, let us worship God.

WATCH OUT! HERE HE COMES!

There is one thing in particular that propels me to worship: Satan. Yep, that's right—Satan. Throughout my journey of faith, I became more aware of when Satan was pushing my buttons. It was often subtle and catered just for my soft spots. Had I not sharpened my sense of discernment and stopped to consider the truth of the matter, I would have dismissed the real source of my distress.

One particular incident comes to mind. I had experienced a glorious day, having attended a women's conference that morning. I was excited to meet my writing mentor, author Edna Ellison, who was a speaker at the conference. To add icing to the cake, Brenda Ladun, a breast cancer survivor was also a scheduled speaker. I had wanted to hear her speak ever since reading her book, *Becoming Better Not Bitter*, which served as inspiration for this Bible study.

Leaving the conference early, I headed to the Race for the Cure event sponsored by the Susan G. Komen Foundation for breast cancer research. My friend Sharon had twisted my arm to walk in memory of her mom. I wasn't sure I was ready, as I was still wearing my wig, but it turned out to be a remarkable event. (You'll read more about it in an upcoming lesson.) When I came home that afternoon, I was approached by a disgruntled neighbor complaining about my barking dogs, which at this point were barking non-stop from his intrusion on our property. He voiced his objections to my dogs' daily welcoming as I pulled into the driveway. Obviously, he felt the need to vent his irritation.

I became upset until I realized "the ploy"—Satan's ploy. I started piecing it all together. First, this neighbor lives two houses down and hasn't talked to me in twenty years. Second, it was broad daylight. Who cares if dogs are barking in the middle of the day? Third, he's a troubled neighbor and has been heard yelling at people and dogs from his deck. Fourth, few things push my buttons faster than bad-mouthing my dogs. Fifth, I had just experienced a moment of a lifetime, so it was the perfect time to crush the "high." Once I considered all these things, I realized there was only one reason why this individual would have accosted me: Satan. Satan wanted to steal my joy. My pastor once said, "Satan wants to steal our joy because he cannot steal our salvation." I confess Satan did steal my joy that day but only for a while. The point is that we need to be aware of Satan's subtle attacks so we can rebuke him and move on.

Recall a specific time when you recognized Satan's intervention. How did you respond?

_____

_____

_____

I'd like to conclude with an original poem written by my friend Sharon Atwood. Let the light seep in the next time you don't feel like worshiping.

Feeling in the dark for the hope in the hopelessness,
the joy in the sadness,
the faith in the fear,
and the light in the darkness.
The tears come, the sadness seems to envelop you.
Look up, look within, look around and see God in all things.
Know that in the crying out, if you listen,
the music of praise from Him will fill your heart.

Open your mouth, open your eyes, open your ears.
Let the hymn of praise be sung and spoken, seen and taken in.
Listen to His praise and let the light seep in.

Meditative Thought

When was the last time you really worshiped God? "I will bless the Lord at all times; His praise shall continually be in my mouth" (Ps. 34:1).

This lesson is dedicated to a humble man of God, Boyd Jordan. He epitomizes the heart of this lesson as he not only continues to worship God through the trials and setbacks of multiple myeloma, but makes the glory of God known to scores of others through his witness.

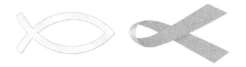

GOD'S PEACE: OUR JOY

Do not be grieved, for the joy of the Lord is your strength.

—Nehemiah 8:10

It was a question I had pondered for months and now it was uppermost in my mind as it was to be the theme for the women's retreat at our church. The theme: Experiencing the Fullness of God's Joy. The question was how was it possible to have joy in the midst of adverse circumstances? Certainly the apostle Paul did. I have also known a few people in my life who did, but it was difficult for me to relate. I couldn't comprehend having that kind of supernatural joy.

I was skeptical as I read about this same kind of joy in Hannah Hurnard's allegory *Hinds' Feet on High Places*. One of the lessons from the Great Shepherd to the main character, Much Afraid, was that "you must accept with joy, all that God allows to happen to you. You must never try to evade it but accept it and lay down your own will on the altar."[7] I was so mystified by that lesson I typed up a summary of it plus a few others and posted them on my refrigerator. *One day*, I thought, *perhaps I can journey to a higher place like Much Afraid and understand and/or experience the truth of those lessons. One day . . . .* Four months later, my journey began.

THE WELL OF PEACE AND JOY

The old hymn "I Am Thine, O Lord," written by the blind composer, Fanny Crosby, in the 1800s, incorporates a significant message. I had missed it all these years until our ensemble was singing a slow arrangement of it. Then, it hit me.

> There are depths of love that I may not know
> Till I cross the narrow sea;
> There are heights of joy that I may not see
> Till I rest in peace with Thee.

There it was—the answer to my question of how it is possible to have joy in the midst of trial. It's in the peace. See it? Joy is a result of the peace I have in God. My focus had always been on the joy, not the peace, which is the underlying root and joy-producer. I'd never considered where the joy was coming from other than God, but it really comes from the peace I have in God which spills over. I envision it as a well: the peace is what is in the well but when the well gets so full it overflows, a change takes place, transforming the peace into joy.

For you to experience the peace *of* God, you must first have peace *with* God. But how do you do that? Again, it's a choice—a choice you must make to boldly exercise faith and trust. It takes a lot of practice to step out; but you will find that peace and joy reside in the security of your faith and trust in God alone, not yourself, not others. "Therefore, having been justified by faith, we have peace with God through our Lord Jesus Christ" (Rom. 5:1). Just as faith and trust lead to peace, which lead to joy, there are two additional accompanying attributes. Read Psalm 28:7 to identify these two attributes.

What are the two attributes? _____ and _____

When we trust in the Lord, He also becomes our strength and our shield. So what is the result of all six attributes combined?

Faith + Trust + Peace + Joy + Strength + Shield = Triumphant heart

FEAR VS. PEACE

When we think of peace, we tend to disassociate it from pain and grief, but that's not a requirement. Beth Moore says, "Peace means the absence of fear and turmoil, not the absence of pain and grief."[8] As a cancer patient, you will experience some amount of pain and grief, but it is also possible to experience peace to accompany that pain and grief. "These things I have spoken to you, that in Me you may have peace. In the world you have tribulation, but take courage; I have overcome the world" (John 16:33). "I have overcome the world"—I love that. Isn't that comforting? I'm so glad Christ has overcome the world since it is evil and full of strife. And if Christ has overcome the world, then He surely has overcome my world of cancer. That gives me encouragement.

Think about how you would rate the level of fear in your life right now at this very moment. Mark it with a circle on the scale. How would you rate the level of peace you have? Mark it with a triangle on the same scale. Next, how would you rate the level of physical/emotional pain in your life? Mark it with an X. And last, how would you rate your level of joy? Mark it with a square.

(O = fear, Δ = peace, X = pain, □ = joy)

Low _____ High

Now let's evaluate your responses. If you have a circle close to the high end, then your peace and joy will likely be on the low end. On the other hand, if your circle is on the low end, then your peace and joy will likely be toward the high end. How does your pain compare to your fear as well as to your peace and joy? Do your peace and joy show an almost equivalent marking on the scale? If not, ask God why you have not experienced the unexplainable joy that comes with His incredible peace. My friend, don't miss the blessings that await you.

DON'T LET SATAN STEAL YOUR JOY—LET IT SHOW! LET IT SHOW! LET IT SHOW!

Throughout my journey of faith, I felt a deep sense of peace, having adopted Psalm 32:7 into my thoughts. "Thou art my hiding place; Thou dost preserve me from trouble; Thou dost surround me with songs of deliverance." I liked the idea of being able to hide in God and be preserved from trouble. It felt secure with God as my refuge. I asked God one day, "How exactly do you preserve me from trouble?" His response: through joy. Perplexed at first by the two-word reply, I quickly realized it was indeed appropriate since I was currently experiencing a phenomenal abundance of joy and was thus being preserved from viewing my cancer as something tragic. This was evident a few days after my diagnosis when I recorded the following in my journal:

> Listening to a CD in my car as I traveled to sing for the morning prayer service, I heard the words to a song about allowing You [God] to control the hard times in life. I thought to myself how I hoped that I would do that when the hard times came. Immediately following that thought it was as if God tapped me on the shoulder and reminded me that I was in "hard times." Chuckling, I admitted, "Oh yeah, you're right."

I had discovered the person, power, and plan of God in my circumstances. I had so much darn joy, it showed in my countenance. People commented on the joy and radiance they could see in my face and eyes. "A joyful heart is good medicine, but a broken spirit dries up the bones" (Prov. 17:22).

But what about when you don't have the joy I speak of? Has it been stolen from you? Did you ever have it? Go back to the root of where joy comes from—God's peace. Find peace with God and you will receive the bonus of joy. Be mindful, though, Satan will steal your joy if he can undermine your peace.

THE JOY BRACELET

Numerous times Satan would creep into my joy and snatch it away. I became more discerning as he got more deceptive. I found myself creating a "joy gauge" of sorts to serve as a reminder of God's joy implanted in my life. One of the love gifts given at the women's retreat I spoke of earlier was a "joy" stone bracelet. During the first few months of my cancer treatments, I wore my joy bracelet every day. The dangling stone bobbled on my wrist, tapping on the surfaces where I was working reminding me all day long of my inner joy. Whenever I felt threatened by Satan's attempts to steal my joy, I would squeeze the joy stone between my fingers as if to say, "Oh, no, you don't." By pressing the stone, I felt as if I were symbolically taking a drink of joy from the flowing fountain of God's river, like a refreshing gulp of lemonade on a hot summer day.

The bracelet had an awkward clasp, making it difficult at times to put on by myself. Some days were harder than others to engage the clasp. I began to notice a correlation between the challenges of the day and the ease of putting on my bracelet. The harder it was to put on, the more I would need to squeeze the stone to endure the challenges of the day and Satan's uninvited interruptions. Silly, I know, maybe even a bit superstitious, but it became a symbolic ritual for me each morning as I began my day with a silent statement of not giving in to Satan's schemes and relying upon God instead.

Is there something tangible that reminds you of God's joy? If so, list it below. If not, think of something (a piece of jewelry, an item of clothing, a writing utensil) that could serve as a "joy reminder."

A Living Stone

One particular Sunday morning I was driving to church by myself since Parker had earlier church business to attend. As I was praising God listening to my CD, a blue flashing light caught me by surprise. I was unaware of my offense, but the policeman said I was speeding in a construction zone area. With tears in my eyes, I apologized not only for my speeding but also for my distraught nature as I had been praying to God concerning my upcoming surgery in a few days. I told the policeman of my cancer and how I had just finished listening to a song that was very meaningful to me. To my amazement, the policeman told me about his mother who was completing her last chemo treatment that week. He wished me well and kindly handed me a warning ticket. (I later wrote him a thank-you note and expressed my joyfulness for his mom. A few days later, I received a card from the officer, wishing me well on my upcoming surgery.)

Satan stole my joy that morning until I realized, as I clinched my joy stone with determination, that I was not going to allow it. I continued driving toward church as I dried my tears. Within minutes, I was stopped again—this time in a long line of traffic. A runner's race was in progress, passing right in front of our church. As I sat impatiently, I reached for some lotion in my purse given as another love gift at the ladies' retreat. I laughed out loud when I saw the name on the tube: "Joy Full" moisture lotion.

When I finally made it to church, I had missed most of the special Sunday school lesson being taught for the women that day. But as they reread the focal verse, my mouth dropped open. "You also, as living stones, are being built up as a spiritual house for a holy priesthood, to offer up spiritual sacrifices acceptable to God through Jesus Christ" (1 Pet. 2:5). "No," I vowed once again, "Satan will not be stealing my joy today." I was a living stone and was being built up to offer spiritual sacrifices acceptable to God. I cherished the thought.

A Lesson Learned

Remember the lessons from *Hinds' Feet on High Places* I posted on my refrigerator? The list remained there for months as I reread it periodically to monitor my progress to the high places. One day I reread one of the lessons and smiled with sheer contentment. Tears came to my eyes as I realized I had somehow miraculously gotten to the place in the midst of my cancer journey that I could say along with Much Afraid, "Behold me, I am thy little handmaiden Acceptance-with-Joy."[9]

Meditative Thought

"The Lord God is my strength, and He has made my feet like hinds' feet, and makes me walk on my high places" (Hab. 3:19). Where are you in your spiritual journey to the high places?

This lesson is dedicated to the memory of Claude Sawyer, who succumbed to multiple myeloma well beyond the usual survival time. He, as well as his family, experienced a roller coaster of emotional and physical trials, yet maintained peace and joy in God's strength.

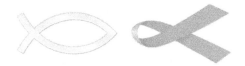

STEPPING INTO GLORY

And after you have suffered for a little while, the God of all grace, who called you to His eternal glory in Christ, will Himself perfect, confirm, strengthen and establish you.
—1 Peter 5:10

We set the stage in the beginning of this study through preparation as we discussed seeking God through His purpose and promises. We confronted the diagnosis of cancer and began processing its impact. We addressed the need for having a medical plan and a spiritual plan. We talked about the effects and changes cancer brings into our lives and relationships. And now we come to the end of the four-week segment of "The Process" in which our responses have been examined. It is in our responses where we discover our strengths, flaws, character, trust, dependence, and discipline. It is here, in our responses, where the impacting differences are found. It is also here where we have the chance to move beyond a tolerance level to a position of glorifying God.

So much is inevitable throughout the cancer journey—doctor appointments, bodily insult, shocks, setbacks, lifestyle changes, loss of control—but as I have said, walking with God and growing through the adversity is a conscious and deliberate decision. Building your faith and worshiping God regardless of your circumstances are noble and worthwhile responses. Finding spiritual outlets of release are also healthy responses. When we make choices like these, we increase our stride. Our steps become surer. We begin stepping into glory, God's glory, a place beyond ourselves, a place beyond cancer. I'm not talking about the glory of heaven after death, I'm talking about the glory found right where you are in the midst of your daily living.

THE "GLORY ZONE"

Being stretched beyond ourselves allows us to operate in what I like to refer to as the "glory zone." In other words, if we are living only in what we can do, then we do not display the wondrous and mighty glory of God through our lives. We need to live and encounter things that we would be unable to do without God's intervention. My friend Gwen is a good example. While going through a stressful job transition, Gwen's confident faith was evident in an e-mail she sent me. Referring to potential jobs, she said, "The darker the place and the greater the challenge, the greater God's light will shine." Gwen lives in the "glory zone." George Brunstad also found his way into the "glory zone." He decided to swim the English Channel at age seventy to raise money for needy children in Haiti. In an interview, he said the purpose for his daring feat was for the glory of God. Not only did he accomplish glory to God, but he also set a world record. His first words upon hitting the sand on the beach of France after the sixteen-hour, thirty-two-mile swim were, "God is good. God is great. Thank you, God!"[10]

Have you experienced a time when you felt you were in the "glory zone"? If so, give a brief explanation.

_____

_____

GLORY REVEALED

So what exactly is God's glory, where is it found, how do we receive it, and what does it look like? Let's start with a description of glory. The *New International Encyclopedia of Bible Words* refers to the glory of God as an expression of His presence both in His people and in the universe. God's glory is rooted in who He is—that is, His very nature, independent of the evaluation of mankind. His glory is found in His splendor displayed through his actions and reflected back to Him as praise. "His splendor covers the heavens, and the earth is full of His praise" (Hab. 3:3). So where is God's glory found? The Bible speaks quite clearly to that. Here are a few examples:

Identify where God's glory is found.

Psalm 19:1 _____

Psalm 66:1 _____

Psalm 148:13 _____

Numbers 14:21 _____

Isaiah 43:20 _____

Zechariah 2:5 _____

John 11:4 _____

1 Corinthians 15:41 _____

God's glory can be found throughout the heavens and the earth, the elements thereof, and the beasts of the field. "For the earth will be filled with the knowledge of the glory of the Lord" (Hab. 2:14). Glory can also be found in sickness. Most importantly, God's glory is found through the death of Jesus Christ, His Son, who brings us salvation. "Therefore we have been buried with Him through baptism into death, in order that as Christ was raised from the dead through the glory of the Father, so we too might walk in newness of life" (Rom. 6:4). It's easy to see—God's glory is everywhere. We expect His glory to be in the sanctuary (Ps. 63:2) and the temple (Ps. 29:9) but not in ostriches and jackals (Isa. 43:20). I've seen God's glory proclaimed through a petting zoo, a man without any limbs, and even a two-legged dog (yes, I said two-legged)!

Not only does God use unlikely places to proclaim His glory, He uses unlikely people. I've heard lots of people reveal their struggle of how God could possibly use them. I have felt that way countless times. The truth is: every person God has ever used has not been perfect or ever will be.

Name three unlikely people in the Bible God used to bring Himself glory.

_____

There are many from which to choose. Your list will be different from mine but I thought of Esther, the Samaritan woman at the well, and Pontius Pilate. Rahab, the prostitute who was in the lineage of Christ, is a good one, too.

God uses unlikely circumstances to bring glory. Cancer or any other sickness demonstrates that. Time after time God's glory is seen through sickness and healing. The centurion's servant in Matthew 8 is an example. "And Jesus said to the centurion, 'Go your way; let it be done to you as you have believed.' And the servant was healed that very hour" (Matt. 8:13). Another example is the leper. "And a leper came to Him, beseeching Him and falling on his knees before Him, and saying to Him, 'If You are willing, You can make me clean.' And moved with compassion, He stretched out His hand, and touched him, and said to him, 'I am willing; be cleansed'" (Mark 1:40–41).

Has God ever used you in an unlikely place or situation? Briefly explain.

_____

_____

_____

When God uses unlikely people in unlikely places through unlikely circumstances, His glory becomes more glorious. Are you getting the picture? "God has every right to exercise his judgment and his power . . . He also has the right to pour out the riches of his glory upon those he prepared to be the objects of his mercy—even upon us" (Rom. 9:22–23 NLT).

GLORY = SUFFERING

We have yet to address how we can receive God's glory. We can know God gives it because the Bible says He does. "The Lord gives grace and glory" (Psalm 84:11). But how do we recognize it? Something we've already talked about: transformation. Transformation of our lives from God's intervention is the indicator. "But we all, with unveiled face beholding as in a mirror the glory of the Lord, are being transformed into the same image from glory to glory, just as from the Lord, the Spirit" (2 Cor. 3:18). Now for the bitter pill, swallow hard. Glory is often received through sharing in the sufferings of Jesus Christ. Paul referred to "the fellowship of His [Christ's] sufferings" in Philippians 3:10. Fellowship? That means Paul + Christ, or a modern day interpretation, you (and me) + Christ. But for us to suffer with Him, Christ first had to suffer. Only then could He enter into His glory. "Was it not necessary for the Christ to suffer these things and to enter into His glory?" (Luke 24:26). Peter reiterates the words of Paul in a letter to the Christians in Asia. They were living and suffering in a pagan society yet remained faithful. "Beloved, do not be surprised at the fiery ordeal among you, which comes upon you for your testing, as though some strange thing were happening to you; but to the degree that you share the sufferings of Christ, keep on rejoicing; so that also at the revelation of His glory, you may rejoice with exultation" (1 Pet. 4:12–13). Did you notice the second qualification of suffering in addition to our suffering with Christ? We should suffer with rejoicing! Could it be any more difficult? Is that possible? As you have already learned, it is indeed possible through Jesus Christ. So it is: we, too, must suffer to enter into glory. "For momentary, light affliction is producing for us an eternal weight of glory far beyond all comparison" (2 Cor. 4:17).

Jesus' disciples counted it a privilege to suffer for their Teacher. Once, while in Jerusalem, the apostles were imprisoned and flogged but "they went on their way . . . rejoicing that they had been considered worthy to suffer shame for His name" (Acts 5:41). Beloved, there's no doubt that you have been suffering in regard to your or your loved one's cancer. It has not been easy. However, I must ask you, have you made the conscious decision to give God the glory through your suffering? You can offer this adversity unto the glory of God and He will use it in unimaginable ways.

What a perfect perspective of suffering Paul gives when he said, "We suffer with Him in order that we may also be glorified with Him. For I consider that the sufferings of this present time are not worthy to be compared with the glory that is to be revealed to us" (Rom. 8:17–18). There it is again—that incomparable glory. I don't know about you, but that verse encourages me and makes my suffering more tolerable. I cherish the thought that if I have to suffer, it can be of value toward the glory of God now, with much more to be revealed to us later.

One last thought before concluding this week's lessons of responses: have you ever thought about what the glory of God looks like? Is it possible to see it or experience it? Yes. The glory of God can come in peaceful ways, thunderous ways, majestic sights, unexpected moments, miraculous occurrences, or in a tender touch. I have seen His miraculous glory in a baby named Miles Darnell. I've also seen unexpected glory in the drowning of a two-year-old child named Bronner Burgess. I've seen it in a falling star following a request for God to show me He was thinking of me. I have heard it in the sound of the ocean waves and watched it in an electrical storm in the heavens. I have experienced it through whispered prayers, visions, meditations, unplanned conversations, and intimate worship. But more than anything else, I have lived in the glory of God by stepping into the "glory zone" while suffering with Him through my cancer journey.

How are some ways you have seen or experienced the glory of God?

_____

_____

One description of what glory looks like is found in the first chapter of Ezekiel, where he describes a powerful vision. "Such was the appearance of the likeness of the glory of the Lord. And when I saw it, I fell on my face and heard a voice speaking" (Ezek. 1:28). Ezekiel's humble response should be reflective of our own every time God pours out His glory. We should soak up His blessings and glory with gratitude, humility, and conviction. C'mon, let's climb the steps to glory.

Meditative Thought

A question posed in the lesson warrants repeating: have you made a conscious decision to give God the glory through your suffering? If not, consider doing it right now.

This lesson is dedicated to the following family members who have stepped into heavenly glory: my aunt Ethel Mae Lankford (leukemia) who portrayed amazing grace to the very end, my uncle Bill Lankford (colon cancer) who persevered in faith, and my uncle Harold O'Kelley (sarcoma) who was a spice of life.

PHASE II

Week 6

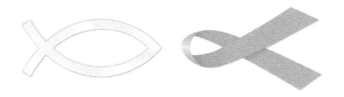

THE AFTERMATH: THE REWARDS

As we enter into the last week of our study, take time to reflect on "The Preparation" and "The Processes" of cancer that have been discussed. While it may not be right now, at some point you and/or your loved one will enter some form of aftermath. I call it Phase II. This is a time when your faith has the potential to become a ministry. As a survivor, it may be the hardest phase, knowing you live in the spotlight of possible cancer recurrence. As a loved one and/or caregiver, you have survived in your own rite and have a story to tell. Whatever your role, reap the rewards of a new faith, a new ministry, and a new you.

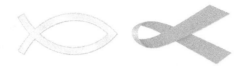

BECAUSE IT'S OVER

This sickness is not unto death, but for the glory of God,
that the Son of God may be glorified by it.

—John 11:4

*O*ver is a relative term especially when it comes to cancer. *Over* can mean sustained life (the cancer is over), it can mark the end of life (a hard-fought battle that is over), or it can mean living in the wake of possible cancer recurrence (over for now). For me, *over* meant an extension of life, a chance to start, well, over. God reassured me early on that my cancer would be healed, my life would go on, and I would fulfill a greater purpose through living. Nevertheless, doubt would creep in time and again, preventing me from fully accepting the message of complete healing. Finally, God revealed it to me in a tangible way.

No More Winters

One chilly evening soon after my diagnosis, I was relaxing in our hot tub on our deck. I was thinking about recent events with a feeling of subdued fear and anxiety when I noticed a large tree. It was early February so there were no leaves on it, only bare branches. I thought of the verse in John 15:5, "I am the vine, you are the branches." The longer I looked at the tree and its branches, the more I began to envision a representation of the human circulatory system with veins, arteries, and capillaries. You remember the pictures in your biology book of the vascular network branching out through the body like a tree? This representation, however, was personal. It was as if the tree branches were my own circulatory system.

I paralleled the nutrient-rich sap pulsing up from the roots into the tree trunk with that of my oxygen-rich blood flowing through my veins into the tiniest capillary. And then something caught my eye: a nest of leaves high in the tree. While it was probably just a squirrel's nest, I saw it as my tumor. I looked at it with awe and sadness. *What does God want me to see?* I wondered. I opened my heart and mind to receive. I began to realize He wanted me to see the tree not only as my body but more specifically as "my winter." I was puzzled at first. It was certainly winter. I considered the seasons of the year and the seasons of life, even seasons of spirituality. Then I thought how grateful I was to at least have the forthcoming joy of spring surrounding me when I went through my chemotherapy. I was thankful I would not have to endure the cold winter months with no hair. I considered that maybe God was telling me this was a season of winter for my life. Yes, that was it. This was to be my season of winter.

Just as clear and calm as those thoughts came to my mind, God allowed me to imagine the tree with green leaves and blooms as if spring had arrived and the tree was full of life again. God impressed upon me that I would see blossoms and sprouting buds; there would be a spring for me and a summer and a fall. There would be no more winters. I interpreted it to mean that life would continue and my cancer would stay in remission. "The winter is past, the rain is over and gone. The flowers have already appeared in the land. Arise, my darling, my beautiful one, and come along!" (Song 2:11–13). Days later, however, Satan cleverly aroused deception within me, causing me to question my encounter altogether. Thoughts of death and defeat snaked its way into my mind. Perhaps I had misinterpreted what I experienced. Perhaps I was being prepared for death just as I had been prepared for cancer, and this would be my last winter. I would have no more. "Trouble and anguish have come upon me, yet Thy commandments are my delight. Thy testimonies are righteous forever; give me understanding that I may live" (Ps. 119:143–144). How could I possibly doubt such real and personal inspiration? I couldn't have made that up. Then I recognized the distortion for what it was. Doubt: Satan's specialty.

Think of a time when Satan has intercepted your thoughts and caused you to doubt what was true. How did you respond? Did you realize what was happening at the time?

_____

_____

_____

THE TORNADO VISION

Cancer patients not only need plenty of support and positive reassurance, they also need a heavy dose of comfort. And so it was for me. Even with the divine revelation of no more winters, I still needed affirmation from the Almighty. *Why am I so resistant? Why can't I just accept God's message to me? Am I that needy I must have further confirmation?* I contemplated. Then I remembered how the Psalms are full of prayers from David needing continuous encouragement from God. David even referred to himself as "needy." I understood. "But I am afflicted and needy; hasten to me, O God! Thou are my help and my deliverer; O Lord, do not delay" (Ps. 70:5).

About a month after the hot tub experience, I was propped up in bed on a Saturday morning having just finished reading a book. I closed my eyes, attempted to clear my thoughts, and wondered how the words I had just read related to my life. An image slowly began to form in my mind. It was an image of a huge glass window. As I focused on the window, I could see myself sitting in front of it gazing out from inside a house. Far in the distance was an approaching tornado. Soon I noticed the wind starting to pick up until it reached a fierce, strong force. The tornado was rapidly moving in my direction. It was a large tornado and was, of course, destroying everything in its path. Debris was flying everywhere as I watched intently through the window in surprising peace and astonishment. As it came closer, a rational thought entered my mind. *This is a tornado, and I'm standing in front of a glass window! I should move away.* I moved toward the door. God told me to open the door and step out, but I rebutted, saying it was peaceful inside and I did not want to go outside with the tornado. Again, I was prompted to open the door. *But why?* Then God clearly spoke to my heart, "Because it's over." I opened the door—the tornado had passed. It was over. I was instructed to go outside and pick up the pieces left behind from the destruction of the tornado's path. I stepped outside and, one by one, I noticed other people coming up behind me until there were many people picking up the pieces.

How would you interpret this vision?

_____

_____

_____

The vision impacted me so profoundly that I was able to squelch any further doubts I had concerning God's message of healing for me. I would survive the tornado (be healed from my cancer), pick up the pieces left behind (restore my life), and move forward (keep on living). I broke down crying and praising God. Soon after, I decided I should call my mother to share the vision with her. Only recently had I begun to understand how traumatic all of this had been for her. I had become so focused on coping the best I knew how that I had failed to comprehend the impact my cancer was having on my loved ones, especially my mother. I was uncomfortable calling since I'd never shared anything like this before with her. How would she perceive it? I swallowed my pride and picked up the phone. After I relayed the vision, she and I cried together as she kept repeating the words, "Because it's over, because it's over." She clung to that for the next six months, telling me several times how much that meant to her and how much hope it gave her. She felt as if God were truly in the midst of her daughter's cancer until it was declared "over" in October 2003 with a negative mammogram report.

What is more amazing is that the vision doesn't end there. Several months later as I was describing the vision to my friend Kathryn, I realized a secondary meaning to the "many people picking up the pieces." I had always thought it strange there were so many people, but now I understood it was meant not only for my support and restoration. Others were picking up the pieces left behind from their own "tornadoes." And now, the truth of that vision lives on through this Bible study. "Record the vision and inscribe it on tablets, that the one who reads it may run [read it easily]. For the vision is yet for the appointed time; it hastens toward the goal, and it will not fail" (Hab. 2:2–3). I am convinced God reveals things to us in stages as we are ready to receive them. We can prepare ourselves by maintaining open minds and keen senses of receptivity.

Numerous characters in the Bible had visions: Daniel, John, Ezekiel, Zechariah, Hosea, and Habakkuk, to name a few. Why shouldn't we in modern times have visions, too? "Then I will pour out my Spirit on all mankind; your young men will see visions" (Joel 2:28). I felt blessed to have been visited by God in such a way.

Have you ever experienced a vision or memorable impression from God? If so, briefly explain.

_____

_____

_____

WINNING THE BATTLE BUT LOSING THE VICTORY

Your or your loved one's cancer trials may not yet be over. In fact, they may just be beginning. Your journey is already proving difficult but victory can be yours. I'm not talking about a guarantee of extended life or the promise that your or your loved one's cancer never will recur. I'm talking about winning the battle in your mind and keeping the victory of faith. Keeping the victory shows what you and I can do; the battle shows what God can do. Warren Wiersbe, Christian author and pastor, warns that the most dangerous time for spiritual attack is when we have won a victory! Did I say, "Won the victory?" That's right. After a victory, we tend to let our guard down and become overconfident, allowing the enemy to move in and defeat us. Great testing often follows great victories. Look what happened to Elijah after the miraculous victory on Mt. Carmel.

Read 1 Kings 18:19–19:4.
What was the victory and what happened afterward?

_____

_____

_____

After the fire from heaven that devoured the wet-soaked wood and oxen sacrifice, followed by the single-handed destruction of 950 false prophets and priests, the victory was lost. Elijah won the battle all right, but he lost the victory. He went into hiding, pleading for death following the mighty battle and great display of God's power. The lesson to be learned is this: Never doubt during the victory what God has taught you during the battle.[1]

THE BEST DEFINITION

Let's tie it all together with one final definition of the word *over*, a definition used by Christ Himself when He said, "It is finished [over]." The fact that He said it brings a whole new dimension to the definition. His death on the cross meant the forgiveness of our sins. His victory over death through His resurrection gives us eternal life. So because it was over for Him (on the cross), it was anything but over for us through His resurrection. To God be the glory.

Meditative Thought

Your or your loved one's battle may or may not be over. Have you been able to pick up some of the pieces the past few weeks through this study? How?

This lesson is dedicated to a mighty prayer warrior, Joanne Campbell, who is well acquainted with God's power. She won her battle with breast cancer and continues to savor the sweet aroma of victory.

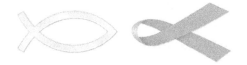

WEARING THE LABEL

Blessed is a man who perseveres under trial; for once he has been approved,
he will receive the crown of life, which the Lord has promised to those who love Him.

—James 1:12

Now that I have entered into the aftermath of my cancer, or what I fondly refer to as Phase II, it comes complete with its own inconveniences and identifiers separate from Phase I. These include continued, but less frequent doctor appointments, diet modifications, scars, bodily tissue changes, weather sensitivity, unexpected flashbacks, daily medication, regimented exercise, prolonged recovery times, new hairstyles, a collection of cancer education material, and a bag full of used wigs, hats, caps, and accessories. Even my mail is indicative of my new label. Yes, I am officially a cancer survivor.

BUT I DON'T LIKE MY LABEL

I am the middle daughter of a middle-class family. My younger sister, Nancy, and I shared a bedroom all the way through high school. My daddy worked long hours as the head maintenance engineer in a nearby paper mill while my mother stayed home and took care of my sisters and me until we were school age. Then she went back to school to complete and expand her college education to become a respected business teacher in the local high school. We lived in the small Alabama community of Sylacauga (sĭl-ə-cŏg-ə), an often mispronounced Indian name meaning "Buzzard's Roost." We ate simple meals at home and enjoyed spending our summer family vacations traveling around the country in our used pop-up camper. I never experienced the stereotypic negativism of being the middle child as I was more than content with hand-me-down clothes, hand-me-down bicycles, and an occasional hand-me-down boyfriend. I wore my labels well: middle child, teacher's daughter, homebody, peacemaker, small-town girl, and Elaine's sister (my older and smarter sister).

But at age 44, I didn't like this new label of "cancer survivor." The title was a constant reminder of something I preferred not to be reminded of. It felt threatening somehow, as if to hold me back from my hopes and dreams. My new label redefined who I was. It also begged the question, "How long will I be a survivor?"

As a survivor I felt obligated to be courageous through any and every trial. But more than anything else, being a cancer survivor identified me with countless other survivors with whom I wasn't ready to be identified. Maybe this was discouraging to me because some of those survivors experienced the cruel re-visitation of cancer. If I simply ignored my current status, could I avoid being one of those second-round survivors? But a nagging and greater question arose: was I unconsciously denying the glory God had in store because of the trials I had faced and now survived? Like the apostle Paul said, "May it never be!" (Rom. 3:4).

Which labels do you willingly carry and which labels are difficult for you to bear?

_____

_____

I vividly remember Nancy telling me as only a little sister could, "Tough, that's what you are now—a survivor. Get used to it." I wondered how she could be so harsh. It jolted me to accept the reality that she was right. I was going to have to find a way to get used to it but how? Certainly God had a plan for me as a survivor. And not just for me but for every survivor.

We confine ourselves when we live within our own expectations rather than being open to adopting God's plan for our future. Look at Jeremiah, the prophet. "Before I formed you in the womb I knew you, and before you were born I consecrated you; I have appointed you a prophet to the nations" (Jer. 1:5). Even before Jeremiah was conceived, God labeled him as a prophet to many nations. Jeremiah 29:11 says, "'For I know the plans that I have for you,' declares the Lord, 'plans for welfare and not for calamity to give you a future and a hope.'" So then, we can surmise from these two verses that not only does God have our future charted before our very existence, but it is one of hope. Are we willing to submit to it? "We may have strong encouragement, we who have fled for refuge in laying hold of the hope set before us. This hope we have as an anchor of the soul, a hope both sure and steadfast and one which enters within the veil, where Jesus has entered as a forerunner for us" (Heb. 6:18–20). Jesus has already gone before us. We need to trust God today for the future He has for us tomorrow.

My Turning Point

I began to soften with my new survivor label at the Susan G. Komen Race for the Cure, an organized fundraiser for breast cancer research. I was still wearing my wig, my scars were half-healed, and my skin was red from the radiation treatments, but I agreed to go on the one-mile walk. I went mostly as a supportive gesture for my friend, Sharon, whose mother had died of cancer the year before. I also wanted Sharon to have the opportunity to express her open support for me.

While at the race I came upon my friend Cathy Munn, who had mentioned to me she would be running for a special friend. I was totally unprepared when she turned around and showed me the sign pinned to her back that read "In Celebration of Karen Allen." I was her special friend! I broke down crying right then and there, succumbing to every vulnerability I had locked inside. Oh, the wellspring of emotions that erupted in those few minutes. It was as if all of my cancer memories converged and climaxed into a sobering and sobbing embrace. I recalled the bodily trauma, the expressions of love, the pain of surgery, the intense sorrow, the overwhelming support, the incomprehensible joy, the day-to-day endurance, the spiritual growth, the embarrassing exposure, the unpleasant side effects, Parker's tears, the disquieting fears, the possibility of death, the bonding of friendships, and the unbelievable nearness of God. It just could not be contained. I cried like an inconsolable baby. Cathy joined me. It was one of the most humbling human blessings of my life. Cathy had made a personal sacrifice to train and run in my honor. She said the three-mile run paled in comparison to what I had been through. As we lingered in our embrace, she helped me understand that I deserved the recognition I was receiving that day. It had been hard to stay spiritually disciplined. How much easier it would have been to give up. There had surely been difficult times, but day by day by day I had placed my focus where it belonged: God.

Read Psalm 121.
How does God respond as you seek His help?

I had chosen not to be identified as a cancer survivor and wear the telltale pink shirt included with the racing fees. I stood on the back row when the survivor picture was taken as if to hide my label. But within hours I was proudly walking down the survivors' "Pink Ribbon Lane" to the cheers of hundreds of bystanders. It reminded me of my high school marching band days as I paraded down the city streets proudly striking my bell lyre amidst the fanfare. Only this time the recognition was for something much more elusive and far more courageous. It was for something I had not stopped to look back on as I had trained myself only to look ahead. But today I gave myself permission to reflect. Today I allowed the mass of support to encircle me with its dynamic impact. Tears streamed down my face as I felt a tremendous outpouring for the victorious battle that had been fought and won not only by me but by every survivor there on that beautiful October day.

I silently bonded with all of the other breast cancer survivors that day, not just at the race in Birmingham, Alabama, but around the country. I permitted myself to become an adopted member of the "cancer survivor family." Each of us had confronted our enemy, planted our flag of victory, and danced around it in joyous celebration. We were a symbol of hope—hope for those who had lost loved ones, hope for those who were yet to be diagnosed, hope for those who were diagnosed with a poor prognosis, and hope for one day finding a cure. All at once the label "cancer survivor" felt right. It felt worthy and noble. The image of being a cancer survivor was changed forever in my mind. It found a home within me—something to be proud of, not something to hide.

Is there a time when your or your loved one's illness helped you connect with others in a more meaningful way? Did it give you increased hope?

The memory of that day will be indelibly inked in my mind—a day culminating in the emotional upheaval of the previous eight months, as if to symbolize I had passed the test. Maybe I didn't cheat death as some do with more advanced cancer, but I had survived the test to become a better person and a better witness. As I slowly completed my walk down Pink Ribbon Lane, I prayed a prayer of thanksgiving knowing it was God—not medicine, not me, not man, but God—who had brought me to this point. And it was God who gave me a memorable and unexpected closure to Phase I, offering it with dignity and grace as if to say, "Here is part of your reward, my child. The rest is yet to come." I accepted the gift with humility. "'Well done, my good and faithful servant. You have been faithful in handling this small amount, so now I will give you many more responsibilities. Let's celebrate together!'" (Matt 25:23 NLT).

Have you ever experienced a time when you felt the reality of the previous verse in your life?

_____

_____

UNEXPECTED OPPORTUNITIES

With my new label came new and unexpected opportunities. Doors began to open. Once I found myself bonding with an older woman in hospice care whom I had been warned might be difficult. With apprehension, I called to introduce myself as her hospice volunteer. When the conversation lent itself, I told her I was a breast cancer survivor. The walls came tumbling down as she began to share freely with me. We visited on several occasions before her death; and I was thrilled to have been able to share some special times with her, particularly with my therapy dog, Frezno.

Another time I was attending a computer training session at work. I noticed a young woman sitting next to me wearing a beautiful pastel pink outfit. During break, we discovered that we were both breast cancer survivors. I openly spoke of how faithful God had been through my cancer journey. She listened with interest.

Time after time, my new label has afforded me opportunities to share my testimony. I have encountered chronically sick people, women with deep personal needs, mentally ill individuals, and people with alternative lifestyles who have listened to what I had to say. God is using unexpected opportunities to manifest Himself through me. I stand in utter amazement at what has happened and what I know is going to come.

ONLY ONE LABEL MATTERS

All of us carry labels distinguishing us from one another. Some labels identify our roles: mothers, fathers, sons, daughters, grandparents, Americans. Other labels are a result of life's experiences: cancer survivor, victim, widow. Some labels describe our unique skills: musician, builder, computer analyst, researcher. Still others identify our character: encourager, motivator, peacemaker, prayer warrior. But when it comes right down to it, regardless of the many labels we carry, there is only one that matters, only one that identifies who we are as believers and seals us with a stamp of ownership. That label is "Christian." It colors all the other labels. Being a Christian establishes our outlook on life and how we live it. Being a Christian determines where our hope lies regardless of our circumstances. And it gives us an eternal destiny with guaranteed heavenly residence.

What are some specific labels that identify who Christ is?

Matthew 16:16 _____

Hebrews 9:15 _____

John 14:6 _____

John 8:12 _____

Psalm 19:14 _____

Mark 6:3 _____

Jesus Christ had numerous labels: Messiah, God's Son, a carpenter, mediator, the way, the truth, the life, light of the world, my rock, my redeemer. All of them distinguished who He was and what He represented.

I am much more than a cancer survivor. I am, more importantly, a Christian, having been adopted into the family of God. If you do not carry the label of Christian, consider exploring its benefits.

Meditative Thought

When was the last time you used the label of Christian to reach out to a seemingly "untouchable" person?

This lesson is dedicated to Patty Lucas and Dale Baldwin, former pet therapy partners. Patty is a breast cancer survivor who always has a kind smile and encouraging word. Dale is a two-time survivor and breast cancer prevention advocate. She wears the survivor label admirably and helped teach me to do the same.

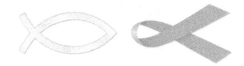

REAPING THE REWARDS

And without faith it is impossible to please Him, for he who comes to God must believe that He is, and that He is a rewarder of those who seek Him.

—Hebrews 11:6

I was a model student. I did my homework every night, studied hard for exams, wrote my own reports, turned in assignments on time, and read the books assigned to me (including Henry David Thoreau). I rarely asked for help on science projects—you get the picture. My dedication and hard work earned me high marks. I deserved to reap the rewards of my labor. Throughout elementary school and high school, ice cream served as a delightful reward, although I was also thrilled with the quarters my daddy gave for each "A." My favorite treat was going to the Tastee-Freez® ice cream shop on report card day. They offered free chocolate sundaes to any student making all A's. Nobody, but nobody, had better tasting chocolate sundaes than the Tastee-Freez®. Each cold and soothing spoonful was pure joy and satisfaction. "There is nothing better for a man to eat and drink and tell himself that his labor is good" (Eccl. 2:24). Anyone for ice cream?

REAPING THE REWARDS: CELEBRATING THE VICTORIES

Rewards are easy to equate in terms of good grades but not so much so in terms of cancer. There were times throughout my journey of faith when rewards served as a welcome break before having to climb the next mountain. Rewards were best accomplished through the celebration of small victories. These celebrations proved to be a vital necessity and were of great encouragement as I progressed through each step along the way.

One such celebration occurred when my chemo treatments were over. The infusion therapy nurses did a song and dance routine in front of everybody in the room. I had anticipated this moment for some time, having observed it for other patients on their last day of treatment. It was a joyful and silly ritual but so wonderfully gratifying after five months of bodily insult. We all laughed and clapped when they finished kicking up their legs and singing.

Sharon and I later celebrated with our own joy dance. We sang and danced around my bedroom like two schoolgirls, jumping, twisting, and raising our hands in praise to God. "And David was dancing before the Lord with all his might" (2 Sam. 6:14). I'm sure our might didn't last as long as David's as we wore ourselves out within a few minutes! We fell on the bed, hearts a-pumping, trying to catch our breath amid the laughter. It was not the type of celebration that could be appreciated by just anybody, but for us, it was the perfect expression of release and thanksgiving. God used those few carefree minutes to unleash months of hopeful concern, giving me a chance to celebrate my victory and Sharon a chance to celebrate life following the pain of her mom's death. "Thou hast turned for me my mourning into dancing" (Ps. 30:11). For my birthday that year, Sharon gave me a ceramic knick-knack of two angels holding hands as if they were dancing. I smile with fond remembrance every time I look at those dancing angels.

Another celebration included ice cream—still one of my favorite treats. At the end of my radiation treatments, the cancer center where I worked hosted a make-your-own-sundae party in my honor. All the fixings were there: three kinds of ice cream, nuts, toppings, sauces, whipped cream, and cherries. It was a sweet celebration with my coworkers to reward my successful completion down the arduous road to cancer treatment finality. I was most appreciative for their recognition of this event in my life.

The best reward of all came three days after my last radiation treatment. Parker and I, along with two other couples, boarded a plane bound for Anchorage, Alaska, to begin a two-week land/sea cruise vacation. The trip had been planned for more than a year and a half, well before my cancer diagnosis. How could we have known the significance of the trip or the timing of it? We didn't but God did. "But if anyone loves God, he is known by Him" (1 Cor. 8:3). We had even changed the departure date at one point to be later than originally planned so we could book rooms with balconies. Had we not done so, my radiation treatments would still have been in progress and Parker and I would have had to cancel the trip. As it turned out, we left right on time and our vacation ended up doubling as a long-awaited reward and celebration.

Have you ever knowingly experienced God's perfect timing in your life? Give a brief description.

———————————————————————————————————

———————————————————————————————————

———————————————————————————————————

The trip was breathtaking with crashing glaciers, vibrant sunsets, diving whales, spawning salmon, pristine snow-covered mountains, and colorful flora. It was nice to soak in the serenity of it all from the ship's deck. The only concern I had was the strong ocean winds. For someone wearing a wig standing on a ship's deck, this had the potential to be disastrous. What if a wind gust came and whisked my wig right into the ocean blue? I laughed at the thought. Nonetheless, I decided to pack an extra wig just in case. Of course it never happened.

The scenario reminded me of another humorous moment when Parker and I went to an elegant restaurant accentuated with soft lights and live piano music. We decided a romantic dinner might curtail our cancer cares for a while. I leaned over the table to grab one of the restaurant's famous homemade rolls. Immediately my silverware snapped to my chest! We laughed as I pulled away the fork and knife from the strong magnets tucked underneath my clothes. My brother-in-law, known by many as "The SuperMagnetMan," had given me the magnets as an added measure of healing. Needless to say, I became more careful around magnetic objects.

SATAN'S PLOY TO DESTROY

The day before we were to board the cruise ship, I discovered to my horror that the zipper pouch containing our tickets was missing. Not only were our tickets missing but so were our passports, $300, a book, and my personal journal—all gone. We frantically retraced our steps, going back to the airport but . . . nothing. We determined it must have been stolen while we were in baggage claim. The passports, tickets, and book could be replaced (and, yes, we were able to board the ship after my angel friend Susan overnighted our birth certificates). Even the money I had planned to use for cruise tips was replaced when I discovered an envelope containing $300 discreetly hidden away by my mother. "And my God shall supply all your needs" (Phil. 4:19). But my journal—my precious journal filled with revelations, intimate prayers, and holy encounters—could not be replaced. It was the documented essence of my spiritual journey through cancer. I had planned to use it as a primary resource for writing this Bible study. Now that hope seemed shattered. How could I possibly remember all that had happened those previous eight months without my cherished journal?

I grieved the loss. How could this horrible thing have happened? "If you are slack in the day of distress, your strength is limited" (Prov. 24:10). I could almost hear Satan laughing at my dismal state of affairs, especially at the impending doom of my unwritten Bible study. I consoled myself by rationalizing that whoever took my journal would at least read some incredible accounts of an awesome God. Not until some time later did it occur to me that God brought something good come out of my calamity. I could no longer be reliant on my journal; I would have no choice but to rely completely upon Him. He would have to bring back to my memory all the things that needed to be said. Isn't that what I should have been doing anyway? Still, in my shaken state, I asked for a sign of confirmation. Within two days, I received an e-mail from my friend, Karen Ott, suggesting that I record my experiences so they could serve as encouragement for others. Karen had no idea I was contemplating writing a book. You are now reading the book I never thought possible after the traumatic mishap in Anchorage, Alaska. "With men this is impossible, but with God all things are possible" (Matt. 19:26).

Describe a time in your life when God took your "impossible" and made it possible.

_____

_____

_____

MY EMMAUS EXPERIENCE

Just as Phase I came with definite closure, Phase II came with a definite entrance. The timing for the Emmaus Walk could not have been more perfect. (See endnotes after Week 1 for an explanation of the Emmaus Walk.) My treatments were completed in August, the cruise was in September, the Race for the Cure in October, and now in November, I was being sponsored to go on the Emmaus Walk, a once-in-a-lifetime event. It marked a time when God would begin to use my journey of faith to reach out beyond my own need to the needs of others. I knew it just as sure as I know my name.

It happened one night during one of the Emmaus Walk highlights as we entered a candlelit room walking through a human-lined winding pathway. Each brother and sister in Christ was holding a flickering candle and singing while waving their hand "I love you" in sign language. There were hundreds of candles illuminating the room. The scene was indescribable. Tears began to flow. As I walked the path, it was transformed into my own Emmaus Road. The symbolism was overpowering. There I was, walking side by side with my teacher down a path of inspirational enlightenment just like the two men on the Emmaus Road who walked with Jesus after his resurrection. "And it came about that while they were conversing and discussing, Jesus Himself approached, and began traveling with them" (Luke 24:15). Unlike these men who didn't recognize Jesus, I knew of my epiphany. Just as the hearts of these two men burned within them as Jesus "explained to them the things concerning Himself in all the Scriptures," (Luke 24:27) my heart also burned within me. "Were not our hearts burning within us while He was speaking to us on the road" (Luke 24:32). Jesus was certainly speaking to me that night, yet not a word was said.

Close your eyes. Imagine yourself on the Emmaus Road. What would you say? How would you respond? How would you feel upon discovering you had walked with the resurrected Jesus?

_____

_____

_____

Phase II had now begun. I was apprehensive but ready. What could I possibly do to help meet the needs of others going through crises in their lives? How could I make an impact on someone during perhaps the most difficult time in their life? I still ask those questions. God shows me every time.

RADICAL REWARDS

Rewards generally have a positive connotation but that's not always the case. I was surprised to discover an alarming number of verses referring to negative rewards. My Deep South layman's definition of *reward* fits quite well: you get what's comin' to ya. Let's look at some biblical examples of negative and positive rewards. "Let him not trust in emptiness, deceiving himself; for emptiness will be his reward" (Job 15:31). Emptiness? I think I'll pass on that reward, thank you. "When one told me, saying, 'Behold, Saul is dead,' and thought he was bringing good news, I seized him and killed him in Ziklag, which was the reward I gave him for his news" (2 Sam. 4:10). Death! So that's where the idea to kill the messenger comes from. "The wicked earns deceptive wages, but he who sows righteousness gets a true reward" (Prov. 11:18). Whew, that's more like it. "The reward of humility and the fear of the Lord are riches, honor and life" (Prov. 22:4). Now that's what I'm talking about. God delights in bestowing the pleasures of reward. Here are some additional verses resulting in positive rewards from God.

Fill in the blanks as to what induces a positive reward.

Proverbs 24:14 _____

Isaiah 62:11 _____

1 Samuel 24:19 _____

Ruth 2:12 _____

Hebrews 10:35 _____

Matthew 6:1 _____

We might expect wisdom, salvation, good deeds, and good works to bring about reward; but we might not anticipate confidence and secrecy to do the same. Now that we've learned some things that bring about positive rewards, let's explore what rewards there are to receive.

Draw a line to match the following rewards with the appropriate verse.

Children	Ecclesiastes 9:9
Enjoying life with spouse	Proverbs 22:4
Riches, honor, life	Matthew 5:12
Heaven	Psalm 127:3

Heaven, life's final reward, an eternal home—what reward could be any greater for the believer in Christ? "Leap for joy, for behold, your reward is great in heaven" (Luke 6:23).

A Thanksgiving Altar

With the recognition of my physical and spiritual rewards, I had a strong desire to give thanks to God for His abundant blessings and remembrance of me during my time of need. Thanksgiving was fast approaching so I decided to create a Thanksgiving altar. I placed several items on it representative of my gratitude, offered a prayer, and lit a candle. It felt right and gave me a chance to commemorate a significant event in my life just as was done in biblical times. "And he [King Manasseh] set up the altar of the Lord and sacrificed peace offerings and thank offerings on it" (2 Chron. 33:16).

In Old Testament times the altar served not only as a place of sacrifice but also as a memorial, reminding the worshiper of a memorable experience with the Lord. One such altar is found in Judges 6 when Gideon prepared a sacrifice of meat and unleavened bread and laid it upon a rock. The angel of the Lord appeared and touched the sacrificial offering with a staff, consuming it by fire. "Then Gideon built an altar there to the Lord and named it The Lord is Peace" (Judg. 6:24). I didn't name my altar, but if I had, it might have been "The Lord Is My Victor." I may not have defeated an army like Gideon, but I sure fought a battle with God at my side to defeat cancer.

Meditative Thought

Have you ever created an altar for a specific purpose? What would you name your altar?

This lesson is dedicated to the memory of my friend Susan Moore's grandmother, one of God's precious saints. Lena Love Patty, who succumbed to myelodysplasia, lived a life of reverent humility until she breathed her last breath in the presence of God and family and went to heaven to reap her rewards.

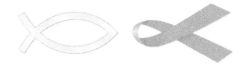

A NEW YOU

Behold, the former things have come to pass, now I declare new things;
before they spring forth I proclaim them to you.

—Isaiah 42:9

In the season finale of *Everwood*, a four-year-running television drama about a neurosurgeon moving to the suburbs, Dr. Andy Brown shares some life lessons at his wife's graveside. "I've changed a lot," he told her. "I've learned a lot. I've learned that what bothers you about your kids is whatever you have in common with them, and what you love about them the most is stuff that you have absolutely nothing to do with. I've learned that pain and suffering are unavoidable but, ultimately, they are what bring you closer to other people."[2] I, like Dr. Brown, have changed, too, and have learned a lot since my bout with cancer. The "old" me is no more; I have become a new person. As Dr. Brown said, pain and suffering have brought me closer to other people.

You have read some of the ways how cancer has changed me, how I evolved through the preparation, the process, and now the aftermath in my journey of faith. You have read my ups and downs, my tears and fears, my joys and triumphs. I have shared intimate thoughts, spiritual encounters, and supernatural reminders of God's presence. I have made myself transparent and vulnerable pouring out my heart with confessions and revelations. Why would I do that? Why would I risk being judged and scrutinized? For one reason: I want you to know how God can walk with you during the crises of your life while at the same time guide you into a deeper faith. I am no different than you in God's eyes, so it is logical for me to believe God can and will do the same for you as He did for me. "For there is no partiality with God" (Rom. 2:11). God uses ordinary people to do extraordinary things every day.

Have you ever done something extraordinary for God? If not, would you like to?

_____

_____

As odd as it may sound, cancer changed my life for the better. I found out what "stuff" I was made of but now there's "new stuff." I'm new and improved. I have a new ministry, a new story to tell, a new outlook on life. I am an example of God's healing mercy and power. I have a new faith, a new perspective, a new voice, and a new song. I like the new me. "I will give you a new heart and put a new spirit within you" (Ezek. 36:26).

I Knew I Was New When . . .

Every morning I take an anti-estrogen pill. I style my (new) short hair and exercise at least three times a week. (OK, I don't always meet that goal, but I try.) My eating habits have changed, my viewpoints have changed, and my relationships have changed. I have developed a fondness for the color pink. Pink ribbons are everywhere—on my coffee mug, my car, my clothing, and my mail. All of these things define the new me, but it doesn't stop there. "Behold, the former things have come to pass, now I declare new things" (Isa. 42:9). I find myself more interested in nutrition, more open to the Holy Spirit, and more compassionate to the hurting. I am more appreciative of life in its simplest form like breathing, walking, and waking up in the morning. I don't take for granted things like hair, eyelashes, and eyebrows. My social pleasantries have expanded as I engage in conversation with strangers about cancer. I've even been known to compare port scars! I find myself creating opportunities to speak of God's love and healing in my life. My corporate worship has been enriched with more anticipation, while my personal worship has become a mandatory need. Music has taken on new heights. I sometimes envision the sound of praise coming from instruments rising up to meet God's ears as He nods with satisfaction. Singing has become a welcome opportunity—no longer a nerve-wracking experience—as I share God's joy in my life. I believe my senses may be keener. Sometimes I detect aromas that make me wonder if I am in the presence of God. "But thanks be to God, who always leads us in His triumph in Christ, and manifests through us the sweet aroma of the knowledge of Him in every place" (2 Cor. 2:14).

Think of some ways how cancer has or might change your daily living and thought patterns.

_____

_____

_____

Cancer tends to prompt one to re-examine not only themselves but their perspectives and priorities. No longer do extra work hours seem so necessary and important. No longer does the sacrifice of time and money for a worthy cause seem so hard to let go. No longer is success measured by what you do and earn but rather by what you have learned and are willing to apply. No longer are relationships of temporal value but are strengthened through the eternal bond of Christian love. No longer are acts of kindness done for the sake of self-satisfaction but are events with eternal significance. No longer is life or the brevity thereof taken for granted but is a daily blessing meant to be lived with fullness in devotion to God. And no longer is the purpose of life questioned but is driven "to demonstrate My power in you, and that My Name might be proclaimed throughout the whole earth" (Rom. 9:17).

NEW-TRITION AND PREVENTION

As a professional in the medical field I would be remiss if I did not elaborate on the hot topics of nutrition, exercise, and prevention. Lifestyle changes are one of the most modifiable aspects to prevention. Don't we all want to know how to prevent cancer and what to do to get our free radicals (cells gone amok) under control? Cancer cookbooks can be found in nearly every bookstore. There are nutrition guides before, during, and after cancer containing unique ideas to ward off the disease. There are antioxidant-rich foods, plant-based diets with low-fat and high-fiber, saturated fat no-no's, red meat and dairy concerns, isoflavins, raw vegetable debates, and vegetarian options. There's salt elimination, avoidance of caffeine, toxin exposure, cooking techniques, food additives, and vitamin, mineral, and herb supplements. I've even seen an endorsement for V8 juice!

Laura Newton, M.A., R.D., a dietitian at the University of Alabama at Birmingham, recommends a wide variety of produce, including deep-colored fruits (grapes, strawberries) and vegetables (eggplants, tomatoes)—particularly cruciferous vegetables (Brussels sprouts, broccoli). These types of foods contain high amounts of antioxidants, which protect against free radicals, making you less vulnerable to cancer. Here is a list of the top twenty most antioxidant-rich foods in order according to the *Journal of Agriculture and Food Chemistry*: red beans, blueberries (wild and cultivated), red kidney beans, pinto beans, cranberries, artichokes, blackberries, prunes, raspberries, strawberries, apples (Red delicious, Gala, and Granny Smith), pecans, cherries, plums, russet potatoes, and black beans.

In addition to being an antioxidant, blueberries, cranberries, and strawberries may also help reduce or reverse declining brain function.[3] So your mama knew what she was talking about when she told you to eat your fruits and veggies. Daniel knew, too. "'Please test your servants for ten days, and let us be given some vegetables to eat and water to drink.' So the overseer continued to withhold their choice food and the wine they were to drink . . . and kept giving them vegetables" (Dan. 1:12, 16).

Read Daniel 1:15
What was the result of a diet of vegetables and water?

_____

Food preparation methods and portion sizes add to the confusion. Where do you draw the line? At one point I started to wonder if cancer was indirectly controlling my life through my food choices. However, a wise friend told me that by making healthy changes in my diet, I was actually taking control so the cancer couldn't. "For you have been bought with a price: therefore glorify God in your body" (1 Cor. 6:20). I did make some minor changes in my diet but nothing drastic. One thing I did was to take a barley supplement for about a year. I don't know whether it helped or not, but it made me feel proactive. I also quit eating yogurt and became more aware of my soy intake. I eat more fruits and berries now and have reduced the amount of red meat I ingest, replacing it with more fish.

Are there some foods you would like to eat more or less of to aid in the prevention of cancer? If so, list them here.

_____

_____

Exercise is as crucial as diet. The benefits of exercise are well-documented. Regular exercise serves not only as a cancer deterrent but also as a deterrent for many other diseases. As Christians, we know our bodies are not our own so it behooves us to consider that in our lifestyle choices. "Discipline yourself for the purpose of godliness; for bodily discipline is only of little profit, but godliness is profitable for all things, since it holds promise for the present life and also for the life to come" (1 Tim. 4:7–8).

Do you exercise regularly? If not, what keeps you from it?

_____

_____

Diet, exercise, maintaining a healthy body weight, and avoiding tobacco are important but are not the only significant factors in preventing cancer or coping with it. As previously discussed, a positive outlook is also very important. A study in Minnesota evaluating the effects of weightlifting for breast cancer survivors revealed not only improved health but an improved outlook on life. Women said they had more strength, speed, and self-confidence. Weightlifting helped them regain a feeling of control of their bodies, reinforcing the benefits of having a positive outlook.

One nonprofit organization for breast cancer survivors in Alabama (no longer active) not only promoted exercise but also adventure. Participants went fly-fishing, horseback riding, mountain climbing, kayaking, hiking, and camping. They professed renewed confidence and spiritual growth. Hence, a positive outlook is advantageous before, during, and after cancer.

I'M READY FOR MIGHTY

OK, we've discussed new lifestyle changes to prevent cancer as well as new physical and emotional benchmarks that may accompany cancer. Now let's zoom in on the spiritual newness you have hopefully gained these past several weeks. "If there is a natural body, there is also a spiritual body" (1 Cor. 15:44). If you have sought God through your pain, worshiped Him through your circumstances, found a joy beyond comprehension through the peace of His comfort, made sacrifices of praise, and confessed your fears, then you have no doubt deepened your intimacy with Jehovah God. I hope this study has prompted you to look inward and seize the opportunity to move beyond your comfort zone. Debby Woods, founder of Racerunners Ministry, says, "I'm sick of comfort zones. I'm ready for mighty."[4] Me too, Debby.

Are you ready for mighty? Are you ready to raise the bar to develop a new relationship with God? If not, what is holding you back? Write your reply so you can see and remember it.

_____

_____

_____

Having read numerous accounts of my unusual symbolisms, I shouldn't have to tell you I was often forced out of my comfort zone. I didn't even mention the time when I gave my testimony and took my wig off in front of the entire church! That was exceedingly uncomfortable for me considering I rarely took my wig off at all. My testimony had a powerful impact that is still talked about today. The bottom line is this: if you are willing to go for "mighty," God will bless it.

My desire is that you have gotten to know God in a more personal way through this study. Only one lesson remains but hopefully you will be able to add to your list of "news," a new relationship with the almighty Father. You may be a seasoned Christian, a new convert, or just contemplating giving Him your heart. Let God work in and through you to develop a new faith. "The Lord's lovingkindnesses indeed never cease, for His compassions never fail. They are new every morning; great is Thy faithfulness" (Lam. 3:22–23).

Meditative Thought

Can the world see a "new" you? Does it bring glory to God?

This lesson is dedicated to Sharon Cummings, my longtime friend of good times past. Parker and I shared many happy memories with Sharon and her husband, Robert, when we lived in Lake Charles, Louisiana, in our early days of marriage. Cancer brought us back together. I celebrate with Sharon the "new" Sharon following her trials with ovarian cancer.

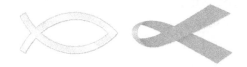

FINDING CONTENTMENT

From the rising of the sun to its setting the name of the Lord is to be praised.
—Psalm 113:3

In the romantic classic *Sleepless in Seattle*, Sam poignantly tells a radio talk-show host how he has learned to cope with life after his wife's death. He explains in simple and honest terms, "I get out of bed every morning telling myself to breathe in and out all day long. Then after awhile I won't have to remind myself to get out of bed every morning and breathe in and out. After awhile I won't have to think about how I had it so great and perfect."[5] It's not ideal, but it works. And what works now will get you to the next step of what works later. Sam didn't plan for his wife to die, just like you or your loved one didn't plan to have cancer; but Sam learned to find contentment in his everyday living. He learned to face the "new normal" in his life.

I fully understand Sam's coping strategy. I felt that way many times. Getting through one day at a time enabled me to get through a week, a month, then a year. Now I feel as if I have a future once again. For a long time I felt as if the possible recurrence of cancer tainted my future. It haunted my thoughts. It is still something I fight against. "But he who listens to me shall live securely, and shall be at ease from the dread of evil" (Prov. 1:33). Like Sam, life seemed "great and perfect" before the invasion of cancer. But because of it, life is different now. I have to find contentment in that. I have to, because God still gives me the ability to get out of bed every morning and breathe in and out, day after day after day.

THE PURSUIT OF CONTENTMENT

When you have what you need, then you will be content, right? OK, then, the real question is, "what do you really need?"

Think about that question. What do you believe you really need to be content?

_____

_____

God's provision is not always the way we imagine it to be, as this e-mail from a friend describes (author unknown):

> I asked for strength and God gave me difficulties to make me strong.
> I asked for wisdom and God gave me problems to solve.
> I asked for courage and God gave me obstacles to overcome.
> I asked for favors and God gave me opportunities.
> I received nothing I wanted but I received everything I needed.

The apostle Paul said, "For I have learned to be content in whatever circumstances I am" (Phil. 4:11). How could he say that? How could he have contentment in prison or after being beaten and stoned? Horatio Spafford, the writer of the hymn "It Is Well with My Soul," said the same thing as Paul. He wrote, "Whatever my lot, thou hast taught me to say, it is well, it is well with my soul." He wrote these timeless words soon after losing his four children in a shipwreck.

Now let's bring it home. Let's just spell it out in black and white: how can you or your loved one find contentment with the looming prospect of cancer in the future? In her book *Calm My Anxious Heart,* Linda Dillow says most of us base our contentment on circumstances, feelings, or other people. However, true contentment is separate from our circumstances.[6] Paul was content because he had learned that the source of his contentment did not reside in an earthly perspective but rather in a heavenly homecoming. He lived with an eternal outlook.

Contentment is a state of the heart, not a state of affairs. Ask the modern-day persecuted Christian. (And, yes, they do exist.) Testimony after testimony is given of persecuted Christians all over the world not only having contentment but having intense joy while suffering for their Lord. Do you think they are happy being tortured? Of course not, but they have learned to separate circumstances of life from contentment with God. The last thing some persecuted Christians want is for others to pray for their persecution to stop. I heard it with my own ears! Instead, they desire prayer for endurance through their difficulties to bring more glory to God. "Therefore I am well content with weaknesses, with insults, with distresses, with persecutions, with difficulties, for Christ's sake; for when I am weak, then I am strong" (2 Cor. 12:10).

Pause for a moment and say a prayer for persecuted Christians all over the world that they may intensify their joy and strength as they glorify God through suffering. (For more information, visit the Voice of the Martyrs website at www.persecution.com.)

What are some things that give you contentment in the midst of crisis?

_____

_____

Philippians 4:11 says, "I have learned to be content in whatever circumstances I am." The word *learned* is significant. Paul had to learn how to be content. It didn't just happen. It took time. I understand that. It took me time. It will take you time. It's a process as well as a pursuit, just like anything else that's worthwhile. Our part in the pursuit is to pray, trust God, and live every day to its fullest measure. Pastor and friend, Dr. Anton Fourie says, "True contentment happens when the things of God become our priority. This coincides with having a proper relationship to God."[7] "For as he thinks within himself, so he is" (Prov. 23:7). What we think shapes who we are. It stands to reason, then, that if God is my priority, He should be foremost in my thoughts. We must take captive of our thoughts—especially if they determine whether or not we are content. "We are taking every thought captive to the obedience of Christ" (2 Cor. 10:5).

Self-absorption is one of the fastest ways to lose contentment. When we think about ourselves, we lose sight of God. Conversely, being within the will and purpose of God is one of the fastest ways to gain contentment. "But godliness actually is a means of great gain, when accompanied by contentment" (1 Tim. 6:6).

DARE TO DREAM

Finding contentment is one thing, but learning to dream again is another. This is a huge step for a cancer survivor—a step demonstrating an act of will that life goes on and is meant to be richly lived day by day and week by week. On the *Comfort of His Holiness* CD (mentioned in "The Shepherd's Comfort" lesson), there is a song that made me cringe every time I heard it. It brought tears to my eyes because I knew I had not arrived yet. The song made reference to dreaming about tomorrow. I couldn't do that. Then one day, over a year later, I came to realize God is already in my tomorrows, and while I may not know what tomorrow may bring, I do trust God. I trust that His plan for me is not yet fulfilled. I trust He will use my tomorrows for His glory if I will allow Him.

> Finding contentment is one thing, but learning to dream again is another.

Here are the powerful words of the song "Candle in the Rain," written by Tony Wood and Mark Harris:

> Heartbreak comes, steals the color from my sky,
> Blue and white fade to black and gray.
> Clouds collide and tears fill up my eyes,
> Storm winds steal the words I want to pray.
> Deep inside of me there is a flame called faith,
> And though teardrops fall, there is a choice I have made:
>
> (Chorus)
> I will dare to dream about tomorrow,
> I will hold to hope through all of the pain.
> I will never surrender to the sorrow.
> No, I will be a candle in the rain.
>
> So I'll go on a light that's burning in the dark
> Reaching out to others all around
> And though lightening strikes and the thunder rolls,
> I have no doubt God is in control.
>
> I will trust that life is more
> Than just what I see before me
> And a bright new day is up ahead,
> Another chapter in the story.[8]

Do you have dreams for tomorrow? If so, list a few.

_____

    I still cry when I hear that song, but now I cry because I can dream about tomorrow and because new chapters continue to be written to my story. Like the song says, sometimes I find myself being a candle in the rain. As Christians, we should adopt that role for the sake of others who need a guiding light. Our flame of faith gives us the choice to hold on to the hope we have in Jesus Christ.

Do you know about the personal hope you can have in Jesus Christ?　☐ Yes　　☐ No

THE MOMENT OF TRUTH

If you answered "no" to the above question, now is the time to get to know that hope. You can learn how to live a fulfilled life and dream about tomorrow. Cancer and this earth are finite; eternity is infinite. Find eternal contentment in the One who died to bring you salvation from your sins. He's the same One who heals your diseases, the One who will never leave you, and the One who hides you under His wing to provide shelter from the storm. He's the One who shines in the darkness and gives you joy through suffering. Will you let Jesus Christ enter your heart right now, this very moment? Will you ask Him to forgive your sins and rescue you from this world of darkness? He can forgive any and all sin, no matter how evil. Will you believe He can save your soul and provide you all the contentment you will ever need? If you said "yes" to any of these questions, tell Jesus right now that you want that. Tell Him you want Him to live in your pain, your sorrow, your hope, your joy, your intellect, your tomorrows, and, most of all, your heart. Let Him transform you into something new, something that will shine through the dark pit of cancer. Remember God is bigger than cancer.

Did you ask God into your heart?　　☐ Yes　　☐ No　☐ I'm already a Christian

    If you asked God into your heart, you have made the greatest decision you will ever make in your lifetime. You should be aware that you will never be the same—and that is a good thing. Please find someone to tell.

LIFE IS WORTH THE LIVING

Throughout this study God has taught me, inspired me, enlightened me, and humored me. He has answered two burning questions for me. The first is: As a cancer survivor, is contentment possible? The answer: Yes, not only is contentment possible, it is profitable because it becomes a testimony of our lives. The second question is: Will I be able to face tomorrow? The chorus of the hymn "Because He Lives" answers that for me:

> Because He lives, I can face tomorrow
> Because He lives all fear is gone;
> Because I know He holds the future
> And life is worth the living just because He lives.[9]

Statements made by two cancer survivors echo my own sentiments, which seem appropriate as we close our time together. Mary Ann Harvard said, "Yes, I have a disease that could kill me, but I am not dead. I feel more alive than ever, and I want to live the best life I possibly can."[10] Lynn Kohlman said, "Every moment of my life is the best part now. I wake up every morning and say, 'Oh, it's so beautiful.' It's not that I didn't appreciate things before, but now I know that life is really moment by moment."[11]

I pose a question to you: How will you choose to live your moments? I choose to accept what God has allowed in the past and what He is allowing today and to give Him all of my tomorrows. Will you do the same? If you can't do that right now, God is patient. He will wait. Ask Him to help you. Pastor B. R. Johnson sums it up nicely by saying, "The One who is taking care of your future is taking care of you right now."[12]

I am going to ask you to do one last thing. Memorize this easy verse. Repeat it over and over and believe it for your life: "Behold, I will do something new, now it will spring forth" (Isa. 43:19). Now go discover what that is.

Meditative Thought

Have you found a place of contentment in your heart? If not, what baby steps can you begin to take in your pursuit? Ask God to show you how and anticipate His response.

This lesson is dedicated to the loving memory of my daddy, George Alton O'Kelley, who has found perfect contentment in his heavenly homecoming with the almighty Father. His encouraging support can be felt even now. Thank you, Daddy angel. I love you.

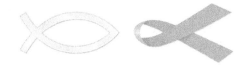

ENDNOTES

WEEK 1

1. Avery T. Willis and Henry T. Blackaby, *On Mission With God: Living God's Purpose for His Glory* (Nashville, TN: LifeWay, 2005).

2. Ibid.

3. Worship.Together.com, featured Worship Leader: Rita Springer, March 1, 2006.

4. Charles Spurgeon, taken from Spurgeon's Daily Devotional, Bible Soft PC Study Bible version 4.

5. Melissa Riddle, "Grit, Grace & Glory," *Homelife*, April 2004.

6. Interview of Mel Gibson by Diane Sawyer on ABC's PrimeTime on February 16, 2004.

7. Warren Wiersbe, *Be Patient: Waiting on God in Difficult Times* (Wheaton, IL: Victor Books, a division of Scripture Press Publications, Inc., 1991).

8. The Walk to Emmaus is a highly structured three-day experience designed to strengthen and renew one's faith and development as a Christian leader. For more information, visit upperroom.org/emmaus.

9. Ken Hemphill, *The Prayer of Jesus: Living the Lord's Prayer* (Nashville, TN: LifeWay, 2002).

10. Shelia Walsh, *Boundless Love: Devotions to Celebrate God's Love for You* (Grand Rapids, MI: Zondervan, 2001).

11. Words and music by Darlene Zschech, © 1996 Darlene Zschech and Hillsong Publishing (admin in U.S. and Canada by Integrity's Hosanna! Music/ASCAP), c/o Integrity Media, Inc., 1000 Cody Road, Mobile, AL 36695. All rights reserved. International copyright secured. Used by permission.

12. Illustration used in a sermon by Dr. Benjamin Littlejohn at First Baptist Church, Birmingham, AL.

13. Sue Monk Kidd, devotional on Someone Cares Dayspring greeting cards, (Carmel, NY: adapted from Daily Guideposts, 1989.

14. Henry Blackaby and Claude King, *Experiencing God: Knowing and Doing the Will of God* (Nashville, TN: LifeWay, 1990, reprinted 1993).

15. Ibid.

16. Words and music by Darlene Zschech, © 1993 Darlene Zschech and Hillsong Publishing (admin in U.S. and Canada by Integrity's Hosanna! Music/ASCAP), c/o Integrity Media, Inc., 1000 Cody Road, Mobile, AL 36695. All rights reserved. International copyright secured. Used by permission.

WEEK 2

1. "What Are the Key Statistics for Breast Cancer?" American Cancer Society; taken from the Internet on June 6, 2008.

2. *Merriam Webster's Collegiate Dictionary*, 10th edition, 1994.

3. Jack Gordon, "Your Friend Needs Help," taken from the Amedisys Hospice volunteer newsletter in Birmingham, AL, January 2005.

4. Nancy Leigh DeMoss, *Brokenness: The Heart God Revives* (Chicago, IL: Moody Press, 2002).

5. Henry Blackaby and Claude King, *Experiencing God: Knowing and Doing the Will of God* (Nashville, TN: LifeWay, 1990, reprinted 1993).

6. "Bring the Breaking" written by Casey Corum, Copyright © 1998 Mercy/Vineyard Publishing (ASCAP), admin. in North America by Music Services o/b/o Vineyard Music USA. All rights reserved. Used by permission.

7. John Franklin and Chuck Lawless, *Spiritual Warfare: Biblical Truth for Victory* (Nashville, TN: LifeWay, 2001).

WEEK 3

1. Adrian Rogers, *The Lord is My Shepherd* (Wheaton, IL: Crossway Books, division of Good News Publishers, 2003).

2. Emile Barnes and Anne Christian Buchanan, *A Tea to Comfort Your Soul* (Eugene, OR: Harvest House Publishers, 2003).

3. Joyce Meyer, "The Power of a Positive Attitude," *Enjoying Everyday Life,* Joyce Meyer Ministries Inc., Volume 21, Number 5, May 2007.

4. *Chemotherapy and You—A Guide to Self-Help During Cancer Treatment,* U.S. Department of Health and Human Services, National Institutes of Health, NIH Publication No. 99-1136, 1999.

5. *Radiation Therapy and You—A Guide to Self-Help During Treatment,* U.S. Department of Health and Human Services, National Institutes of Health, NIH Publication No. 01-2227, 2001.

6. Taken from the article "As the Clock Ticks Down: Alumna Makes Unique Campaign Gift" published in *The Talon*, a University of Southern Mississippi Alumni magazine.

WEEK 4

1. Susan Cambria, "There is No 'Right Way' to Have Cancer," *Cure*, Fall 2002.

2. *Understanding Breast Cancer Treatment: A Guide for Patients*, National Institutes of Health, National Cancer Institute, NIH Publication No. 98-4251, reprinted July 1998.

3. Television interview by Mike Royer on NBC, re-aired on May 14, 2004. *"Spirit of Alabama"* special segment "Radical Trust."

4. CBS 1994 television series *Touched by an Angel*.

5. Ken Hemphill, *The Prayer of Jesus: Living the Lord's Prayer* (Nashville, TN: LifeWay, 2002).

WEEK 5

1. Victor Parachin, "Dealing with grief," *The Alabama Baptist*, December 9, 2004.

2. Article written by Scott Adamson "Fighting Sullivan" in the *Birmingham Post-Herald*, December 23, 2004.

3. Beth Moore, *Living Beyond Yourself* (Nashville, TN: LifeWay, 1998, revised 2005).

4. Personal e-mail received from Dr. B. R. Johnson on October 3, 2003.

5. Marilyn Meberg, *Boundless Love: Devotions to Celebrate God's Love for You* (Grand Rapids, MI: Zondervan, 2001).

6. Lawrence O. Richards, *New International Encyclopedia of Bible Words* (Grand Rapids, MI: Zondervan, 1991).

7. Hannah Hurnard, *Hinds' Feet on High Places* (Wheaton, IL: Tyndale House, Inc., 1975).

8. Beth Moore, *Living Beyond Yourself* (Nashville, TN: LifeWay, 1998, revised 2005)

9. Hannah Hurnard, *Hinds' Feet on High Places* (Wheaton, IL: Tyndale House, Inc., 1975).

10. Article written in *Partners* magazine, "Still waters run 'deep' for this English Channel swimmer" (Nampa, ID: Aim Companies, Jan–Feb 2005).

WEEK 6

1. Warren Wiersbe, *The Bumps Are What You Climb On* (Grand Rapids, MI: Baker Book House Co., 1999).

2. ABC 2002 television series *Everwood*.

3. *Journal of Agriculture and Food Chemistry*, June 2004.

4. Bible study led by Debby Woods, founder of Racerunners, a non-denominational, evangelical Christian ministry established in 1984.

5. *Sleepless in Seattle* is a romantic comedy/drama movie released in 1993.

6. Linda Dillow, *Calm My Anxious Heart* (Colorado Springs, CO: Navpress, 1998).

7. Taken from a sermon by Dr. Anton Fourie at First Baptist Church, Birmingham, AL.

8. "Candle in the Rain" written by Tony Wood/Mark Harris, Copyright © 2003 New Spring, Inc./Row J, Seat 9 Songs/Ryanlynn Publishing. All rights reserved. Used by permission.

9. "Because He Lives" words by William J. and Gloria Gaither. Music by William J. Gaither. Copyright © 1971 William J. Gaither, Inc. All rights controlled by Gaither Copyright Management. Used by permission.

10. "Living with Cancer" article published in the *UAB Crossroads* magazine, 2006.

11. Article published in *People* magazine, September 19, 2005.

12. Taken from a sermon by Dr. B. R. Johnson at the Lighthouse Community Church in Harpersville, AL.

Did this book touch your life?
The author would enjoy hearing from you.
Contact her at Karen@confrontingcancerwithfaith.com
or write her at:

Karen O. Allen
5101 South Broken Bow Dr.
Birmingham, AL 35242

To order additional copies of this book, visit
www.confrontingcancerwithfaith.com.
Also available in e-book format.

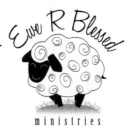